MW00823840

MAN CAVE

OF HEALTH

A Why-To Book About Men's Health:
Through The Eyes of a Health Coach
Who Has Heard It All

LARUE PALMER

Copyright © 2021 LaRue Palmer

All rights reserved

No part of this publication may be reproduced, distributed, or transmitted
in any form or by any means, including photocopying, recording, or other
electronic or mechanical methods, without the prior written permission
of the publisher, except in the case of brief quotations embodied in critical
reviews and certain other noncommercial uses permitted by copyright law.

The resources in this book are provided for informational purposes only
and should not be used to replace the specialized training and professional
judgment of a health care or mental health care professional.

Neither the author nor the publisher can be held responsible for the use of
the information provided within this book. Please always consult a trained
professional before making any decision regarding treatment of yourself or
others.

ISBN: 978-1-7373412-0-8

Published in 2021 by LaRue Palmer

LARUE PALMER
– HEALTH –

To contact the author for speaking engagements or signed copies, email:
larue@laruepalmerhealth.com

Credits:
Cover and Interior Design: Deborah Perdue
https://illuminationgraphics.com
Editor: Margaret A. Harrell, https://margaretharrell.com
Illustrator: Teddy the Dog, https://teddythedog.com/?rfsn=3270583.51d22e

Dedication

To the memory and legacy of my parents,

Jonathan and Geraldine Palmer, who for the

short time they lived on this earth were able to

give me a strong foundation which has enabled

me to speak truth to culture. Throughout my life

I've done my best to make you proud, and to

leave the world a better place.

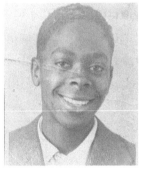

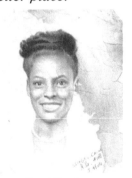

Jonathan B. Palmer
1929 - 1966

Geraldine Lee

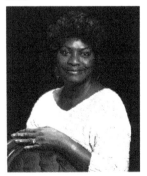

Geraldine Lee
1929 - 1990

Acknowledgments

To my wife Ziva, who believed in me long before I believed in myself. Thank you for being my #1 cheerleader, supporter, and advisor. I love you! And to my daughter Arielle. Thank you for your undying faith in me. Continue developing your brilliant mind, and I hope I've set a good example for you to follow.

To my eldest children, Jevon, Eyvette, Nikiya, and my beloved grandkids, my extended family, friends, and especially those in the Body of Christ, I am indebted to you for affirming that I should carry this important message of men's health to anyone willing to listen.

Contents

Introduction

Every guy knows what a man cave is, right? You might even have one yourself. Chock-full of your favorite man toys, creature comforts, and a well-stocked cooler. It's your special place. It represents that space men like to withdraw to for refuge or recreation, where you can clear your head or just unwind. An escape.

It's in a man's nature to escape at times, because many of us need that separation in order to solve problems swirling around in our head. It's a good thing to get away and clear your head, let off a little steam, or regroup, then get back in the game. Women are different in this respect: they solve problems—at least, personal problems—by talking through them, while men tend to do the man cave thing. But too many of us escape responsibilities by defaulting to our man cave, and that wreaks havoc on many fronts.

As a health coach I've seen this default choice affect men very negatively, when they are facing health issues and do the man cave thing—by not going to the doctor, not telling their spouse or friend. Getting depressed about it, they go even deeper into their cave.

In this book I've reimagined the man cave to include wisdom and companionship, instead of just solitude. In your cave (virtual or physical), you need someone who will encourage you to get help when you need it, or make your own appointments to see a doctor on a regular basis, whether you're afraid or not. Through my life experience of dealing with my own sometimes life-threatening health issues, I'll give you a perspective that even I never expected, where I had to face my own fears. But face them I did. And I'll share experiences of men I've encountered in my practice that will hopefully serve as a wakeup call to be more responsible about your health and why you should be.

Man Cave of Health is not so much a how-to book, but a why-to book. It will challenge you to think through your "why," as in why you should get deadly serious about your health, especially as you age. At sixty-eight, I've been blessed with relatively good health, and a positive aspect about life that motivates me to sustain my health span as long as my life span. I want to project that mindset onto you. If you have a family, they want to project that mindset onto you too.

Between you and me, I see myself as part of an endangered species. That's right, men are an endangered species when it comes to quality of life and longevity. And it's not just by virtue of being a man. We make bad decisions, lots of them, and they endanger our well-being, as you will read in the coming pages. What's disheartening is that most of the warnings that go out to the men I encounter in my profession go unheeded. But still I persist, because I get it.

There's a vestige of a scared little boy running around inside most of us. And when pressed to be a man, we want to run and hide in our little cave. The fact that women on average live five years longer than men should bring you running and screaming out of your man cave, but it doesn't. We think if we hide out long enough, the problems we face as we age will go away. But they won't. Someone will eventually have to go into your cave and carry you out on a stretcher if you're not wise.

CHAPTER 1

The Boy Becomes a Man

A Dysfunctional Role Model

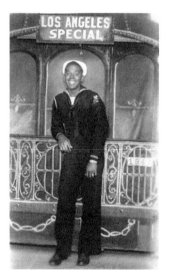

My father, J. B. Palmer

The brief life of J. B., as he was known, ended at age thirty-six. That was my dad, Jonathan Buster Palmer, pictured in 1947 at age eighteen in the prime of life, serving his country as a US Navy sailor in the postwar Pacific. It is heartbreaking to realize that at the time the snapshot was taken, he had already lived half his life. But his untimely demise would end up having a positive ripple effect, encouraging me, his eldest son, to make better choices. When I grew into a man, I resolved to live my life being present with my family—the antithesis of what my dad's life became.

Dad made some excellent choices. For starters, he married my mom! Sadly, the excellent choices effectively end there. J. B. was a talented trumpet player, a loving husband and father, and he had a free spirit with an amiable smile. Many loved him, but he did not seem to love himself, struggling with feelings of inadequacy which he tried to exorcise with alcohol. That was a terrible choice. It would get to a point where Dad ran out of choices.

As a Southern boy, young Jonathan was raised in Atlanta, Georgia, by his two deeply religious parents. Family life revolved around the Baptist church, and they were close-knit. The Palmer household was multigenerational, with my paternal great-grandmother Melinda and my grandfather's sister, Mary Brigham, both living under the same roof. My grandfather Milton was a farm laborer, who served in the army during World War I. My grandmother Fannie worked as a cook for a private family for a number of years, to help make ends meet.

Life was hard, so the family grew much of their food in their backyard, and raised chickens as well. When they migrated to Los Angeles from Atlanta, they continued their urban-gardening tradition. They even raised chickens in their backyard in Watts, California, at the very center of what became ground zero for the Watts riots decades later. My favorite memory of my grandparents was visiting their home and enjoying canned peaches from their peach tree.

Mom always prepared healthy meals. I was often her little side-kick in the kitchen, asking lots of questions. I recall how I used to pretend I was a chef, making scrambled eggs and sugar toast! It was not too many years later that Mom started declaring I was the best cook in the house. I preferred her cooking to mine, but the challenge of trying to duplicate what she did in the kitchen set the tone for me to ultimately become an immensely accom-plished chef. Mom always added a touch of love to her food, which I do to this day!

But it did not take long for my family's quality of life to take a nose-dive. Thanks to Dad's alcohol abuse and sexual promiscuity, some days food was scarce. Each incident of domestic unrest, stemming from yet another drinking binge, further diminished any hope of stability. I even witnessed Dad physically abuse my mom by stab-bing her in the face with a pair of scissors. And at seven years old, as she confided in me what she was going through, I became her unwitting bedside psychiatrist. She would come into my room at night when Dad was out drinking and just start talking to me about her troubles. Trying to stay awake and alert, I would fade in and out, picking up key words instructing me to continue loving my dad despite his shortcomings. I am convinced that she used secret military brainwashing tactics to make sure I never repeated the same mistakes. I can still hear her voice from those bedside chats today, even though she has gone home to glory.

My dad struggled with his demons; his life was spiraling out of control. Eventually, as he lost many jobs and friends, his behavior led to a separation, something I had always dreaded. One fateful day after work, my dad stopped at his favorite bar and got severely intoxicated. I remember it was a Friday, so he had probably just cashed his paycheck and went to tie one on. Another one of those bad choices that I told you about was getting in his car to drive home. This was the time before seat belts, much less mandatory seat belt laws, and in those days they made cars of steel and chrome, not plastic and aluminum. Despite this, his car was totaled, and he suffered massive injuries, mostly from the steering wheel. The police report said he must have been traveling at a high rate of speed when he had a solo accident on a remote road, hitting a tree head on, then a telephone pole.

The doctors did not expect Dad to survive the night, yet he survived six months in a quadriplegic state, in a coma most of that time. One day while Mom was visiting him in the hospital, my dad experienced a significant change in his condition. Mom saw tears streaming down his cheek as he began to come out of the coma, a couple of months before his thirty-sixth birthday. Apparently, he was moved to tears upon hearing my mom tell him I had fashioned and tooled a fine leather wallet for him by hand for his birthday. Once he was completely out of the coma and alert, the horror of his condition set in, and his crying increased to where they had to clear his tubes and calm him down. His wife, the woman he did not feel worthy to have, was faithfully by his side, sharing the fact that his kids all missed him.

Stepping into Manhood

When I turned thirty-six, I too had three beautiful children and a wife. Having reached that milestone, for the first time I had some perspective on what it might have felt like for my dad to be lying on his deathbed, realizing what he had done with his life.

In the end, he could only cry. He was bedridden, totally paralyzed, unable to speak to or even hug his family and tell us he was sorry. On August 3, 1966, Jonathan Palmer died alone in a hospital in the middle of the night from pneumonia, and a broken heart.

This personal glimpse into my life gives you a clue into what motivates me to speak boldly to men about some important areas of their behavior. As a health coach, I am privileged to have grown-up discussions with men who might be on a similar path of self-destruction but in a different way. Engaging in candid discussions with men about their health can be a challenge because men would much rather avoid the topic, especially if they are already seeing signs of physical decline. They want to hide things from me because they are embarrassed and secretly afraid.

What they don't realize is that I already have a good idea what they might go through, because the symptoms men experience past a certain age are so predictable, especially when they voluntarily give me clues without realizing it! With my interviewing skills I'm able to discern if a stressful job or calling might be taking a silent toll on a man's life and how I can alleviate that situation.

Men have a very particular way of finding the right motivation. Dire warnings about future health problems are not an effective motivator. Most humans are "present biased"—and men especially. We have a knack for compartmentalizing, and as long as there's no immediate danger, it becomes a case of being out of sight, therefore out of mind. If a health scare grabs a man's attention, or perhaps a doctor's warning, then fear becomes an effective tool. But there are millions of men in the US who have mastered the game of self-deception. Don't believe me?

Just look at how the clothing you see some guys dressed in, in public! It has become a kind of fashion statement to wear clothes that cover up the *Dad bod!* In addition, men are often tight-lipped about aches and pains they're suffering with. They typically won't speak to other men about their health concerns or fears and even try to hide symptoms from their spouse. Fortunately, a good many women are too perceptive to be fooled by this. I married one, so I know all too well.

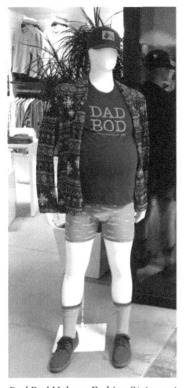

Dad Bod Makes a Fashion Statement

We men don't want to make a big deal out of anything related to our health. We say things like, *"No need to sound the alarm!* Or *"It's not that big of a deal!"* I've heard them all, some as recently as yesterday. Part of the psychosis of men is to pretend that we've got everything under control. We don't want to give up thinking we are in control, even when we know we are not. It's a man thing!

I have heard men say in different ways that the threat of imminent death was the only thing that would get them to finally break down and go to a doctor or hospital, and if they wait till then they'll be in great distress certainly. They can play the eternal tough guy act only so long, and then the body must collect on the debt. I enjoy working with a man who has a personal sense of motivation to reach his health goal because it's usually something close to his heart that provides real motivation.

I'm speaking of the man who might know his youngest daughter's soccer team will be looking for a new assistant coach in a few months. He has missed coaching ever since his oldest daughter stopped playing a few years earlier. Now he wants to put his hat in the ring for that coaching spot, but he's fifty pounds overweight and out of shape. There is no way he could keep up with a herd of teenage girls running up and down the field while carrying that beer belly around!

As his health coach, I see this as my golden opportunity to tap into that motivation in order to get him to get in shape. It's rare that I come across people who can, through sheer will, drop fifty pounds by following everything I tell them to do. We're all flawed in our humanness, so we negotiate with ourselves. By under-standing that, I can apply the appropriate amount of pressure when necessary. I can recognize the potential here for this dad to put in the work necessary to take the excess weight off, based on his stated goals. His "why."

In this situation, I'm just playing a supporting role. Getting his BMI into the normal range because his doctor said he should does not motivate this guy, but fulfilling a dream to coach his daughter's soccer team one day does. Plus he wants to make his daughter proud because he's an excellent coach. He's coached many championship teams before.

A doctor telling him to reduce his weight, as his blood pressure and blood sugar are high, doesn't move the needle, even though it should. It would motivate me, but that's just me. I have to find his pain point, the one thing that triggers his masculine drive to win.

The fire burning inside me to stay vital and active in life led me to leave my career as a leading chef and become a health coach and diabetes-education specialist. I know full well the cost of making poor decisions firsthand, and my heart breaks every time I learn of a preventable situation that became worse because of a delay in getting treatment. If I'm being honest, I can admit to my own tendency to procrastinate in addressing health issues. I can also admit to feeling a foreboding sense of fear of finding out I have a serious health problem in the past.

But I will default to my desire to know what the issue is and *what it will take to resolve it*, which overrides the fear. Having a fatalistic attitude about any health concern is not healthy, especially when it could be something treatable. Once we create our own self-fulfilling prophecy of doom by not taking action, we've diminished our chances of having a positive attitude, which is essential for healing and recovery.

Life can get in the way so easily; then one thing leads to another. You miss one doctor appointment, then the next, and the art of rescheduling becomes a personal pastime. If you have symptoms worthy of looking into, like urinary pain or discomfort, you wait and hope it will pass, or you might even try some over-the-counter remedy. Your remedies might work for a while, so you continue to hide, but gradually your symptoms worsen. Now you are worried, paralyzed with fear. Believe me, I know the drill because I've lived it! I'm just not as stubborn as some men are.

There was a time when I went years with no concern to go to the doctor for a physical, or even the dentist! When I broke down and went to the dentist, I had ten cavities, and I had never experienced a toothache. That was an early sign that if I let things run their course, my body will continue breaking down as the years roll by. When I finally got a general checkup and it turned out my vitals were good, I was greatly relieved, but I was sweating bullets waiting for the lab results.

Getting older is inevitable, but I'm determined to live my life as vigorously as my health will allow at every stage, and I intend to take as many men down that same pathway to optimal health as I can! At the time of this writing I'm sixty-eight years old, recovering from Stage 1 bladder cancer, and I feel blessed to be feeling energetic and physically fit. Because of my relatively good health, I'm kicking cancer in the ass! And you best believe I'm raising the bar on myself to get even better. Cancer develops over years, and you can't avoid everything—stuff happens. The question is, what are you going to do about it? Like I always say, you only get one life to live. Live it the best way you can. My buddy Adam Baker lives with Type 1 diabetes. Years ago he told me, "LaRue, I kid you not, if it weren't for this diabetes thing, I wouldn't be as healthy as I am right now." That statement means more to me today than when I first heard it.

I decided a long time ago to be proactive. My goal is to prolong my *healthspan* to last about the same length as my *life*span, and I am telling you, yes TELLING you, *that's what's up!*

As you read further, you'll learn how most people spend the last twenty years of their life with multiple chronic diseases, treating *only* the symptoms. Those diseases will continue to worsen and ultimately kill them. Yet, *most are preventable.* Even if you land in the hospital, you should do everything to give your body the best chance to fight whatever illness you're facing. When you're taking a bunch of pills to treat the symptoms of high blood pressure, diabetes, or high cholesterol, you're not fighting anything. You've already lost. Big Pharma has won, because your doctor is going to be pushing pills at you until you die, and they will probably add a few more to your pile before you're gone. Most drugs don't cure you of anything; drug manufacturers intentionally design them to just manage the symptoms and keep you coming back for more. By now, you know that the Western medicine model is disease-based, rather than prevention-based. So its primary goal is to treat symptoms of disease and not their cause. If Covid-19 taught us anything, it's that our body's immunity is our best weapon. We'll talk more about that later.

In the US, 58 percent of the victims from the pandemic were men over the age of seventy with preexisting conditions, according to CDC statistics. There's no reason to think there will never be another pandemic, so it behooves us to be prepared for the unknown by maintaining a strong immunity to disease.

A Perfect Example

One thing you will learn about me fairly quickly is that I'm a straight talker, and I don't beg and plead with a client. They pay me to tell them the truth, much of which they already know. I'm there to remind and sometimes nag them. I'm just the guy that's going to keep them on program. So I focus on reminding them that the primary responsibility for their health rests with them. I'm telling you the same thing. You are the main man in charge of your health. Let me share a personal story to show you what I mean.

Just as the Covid-19 pandemic of 2020 happened, I began experiencing a frequent, urgent need to urinate both day and night. I always get up at least once or twice during the night to pee, which I've been doing for years. But this was way more frequent, sometimes four or five times a night. And during the day the frequency was getting ridiculous, notwithstanding the fact that I drank a lot more water than the average person. Sometimes I would sit for too long in one sitting. Then when I stood up, I had to rush to the bathroom.

As the pandemic progressed, it was clear there was more going on than what I suspected: A urinary tract infection (UTI). My wife has some experience with UTIs, so I know a little about them. Just enough to be dangerous. In my mind, I kept saying to myself, *I'll go to see Dr. Stone* ("Stoney," as I called him!) *and get some antibiotics as soon as this Covid lockdown eases up.* Hospitals were bursting at the seams, and news reports made me disinclined to go rushing into an overcrowded medical facility's waiting room, just to check out this *minor* problem. Besides, the authorities were telling everybody to shelter in place. A convenient excuse in my case. So I—along with millions of other Americans—let my medical condition go untreated.

Out of nowhere, I started seeing a slight discoloration in my urine. A little darker than usual, more of a faint copper hue, which was weird. Then one day what looked like a tiny red blob plopped out of me, dropped into the toilet bowl and sank. It was a blood clot. I wasn't sure at first what it was, and I certainly didn't know what it meant, but it got my attention! I even took a picture of it. Weeks went by and there were no new signs of blood clots, and the discoloration was off and on. By now I was boosting my intake of water and cutting out all beverages except coffee. As the weeks rolled, my symptoms worsened, until the water in the toilet after I peed was the color of Dr. Pepper.

Using telehealth with my clients is quite common for me. I often explain the technology, assuring them I use a proprietary, secure video platform that is HIPAA compliant. Now that we've entered the age of Zoom calls, television shows like *Chicago Med* are even depicting these sessions! So, I used telehealth on myself to sort out this growing mystery. I got in touch with a doctor on call because Dr. Stone was on vacation. He instructed me to go to my local lab and get a blood panel and urinalysis done.

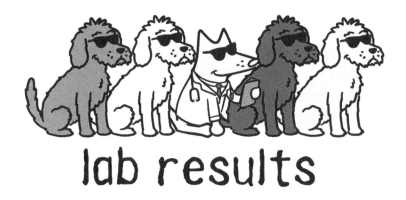

lab results

In a few days, my results were back, and they popped positive for cancer but were "inconclusive" as to what type! Inconclusive? I was confused. I popped positive for cancer, but the doctor was not sure where it was located or the extent, so he didn't want to commit to anything. He urged me to consult with my regular doctor on his return. A few days later, Dr. Stone was back from vacation. I went to see him, and he gave me a thorough physical, including an extensive blood panel and urine screening, then referred me to a urologist he worked with on a regular basis. Before I met with the urologist, I needed to get a CT scan. The day of truth finally came when I would meet my urologist, Dr. Gupta, who was going to give me the scoop.

On November 20, 2020, my wife, Ziva, and I sat in Dr. Gupta's office at Cedars-Sinai Hospital in Los Angeles, awaiting my first consultation. Dr. Gupta had slides from the CT scan revealing a tumor on the inside of my bladder wall. The exciting (kidding!) news was that he was going to perform a cystoscopy on me that day. The exciting (still kidding) part was that I was going to get to see my tumor on a monitor! One of the biggest man-up moments in my life was when I had to lie back and allow Dr. Gupta to insert a catheter-like instrument called a cystoscope into my urethra (the place where only urine flows out!) and up into my bladder, so that the camera on the end of the cystoscope could see inside my bladder.

I imagined the experience to be far worse than it ended up being. By now millions of men have survived multiple cystoscopy procedures and lived happy, productive lives. When I looked at the screen to see inside my bladder, it was like watching a black-and-white version of *Voyage to the Bottom of the Sea*. The cystoscope comes equipped with its own flowing water, waterproof camera, and lighting! You've heard of out-of-body experiences? Well, this was my inside-the-body experience!

With the informative demeanor of a deep-sea-diving instructor, Dr. Gupta proceeded to give me a video tour of my bladder, pointing out a small white growth that seemed to be growing on an ocean floor. Then, the gracious tour guide that he was, he showed me the right side, which had no tumor, so I could see the difference. I was understandably a little freaked out by this mechanical probe way up inside me, so I thanked Dr. Gupta for his expert maneuvering and asked if he wouldn't mind wrapping it up and getting that thing out of me!

When the bladder tour was over, Dr. Gupta informed me he would be using the same type of device for my minimally invasive surgery, but with different attachments to scrape out the tumors and remove them. Only, this time I would be asleep. I appreciated the fact that my surgery would be minimally invasive, because by the time you read this I will have had three of them, with no scars on my body!

Ziva sat through the entire procedure with me, and I didn't say this then, but she looked a little green around the gills. After I got dressed, Dr. Gupta wanted to schedule my surgery. Given that the Thanksgiving holidays were upon us, he suggested we wait till afterward, giving me an opportunity to spend some quality time with family. Without even looking at Ziva I asked him, "When is your very next available appointment for surgery on your calen-dar?" He said November 25, one day before Thanksgiving Day, which was only five days away. "I'll take it!" I said.

In my mind, there was no better time than the present to move forward. I remember being very calm the day of my surgery. Dr. Gupta visited me in the pre-op room early that morning and reassured me he would take good care of me. It was a four-and-a-half–hour procedure, and a success! I went home that evening, relieved that the process of recovery had begun. The next day we had an uncommonly quiet Thanksgiving Day. Usually, I'm cooking for thirty to forty friends and family. To be honest, I didn't realize we were breaking an eighteen-year-old tradition, but it would have been broken anyway, due to the Covid lockdown. On my birthday, the next day, my friend and partner in the health industry, Dr. Tyra Beavers, blessed us by delivering a complete turkey dinner with all the trimmings. I'm both a chiropractic patient of Dr. Beavers and a partner in her clinic as a health coach, and here she was still caring for me. She and her husband Don waived to me from our front door, wearing their face masks, as I lay in full recovery mode on my recliner sofa.

Obviously, I never counted on any of this happening to me, especially in the middle of writing a book about men's health and how men don't take care of their health but choose to avoid regular doctor visits. It became clear that God thought my book needed more of a personal journey to bring my talking points home! I became a living example of what to do when something is not right with your health. In my wildest dreams, would I ever have thought I'd be written into the script!

So, the long and the short of it is this. Following my surgery to remove what turned out to be four tumors from my bladder, the biopsy confirmed that I had Stage 1 bladder cancer. Now, just think if I had ignored my symptoms. I would have ended up like any of the guys I've heard from since my ordeal, some of whom had to have their bladder and prostate removed because they waited too long. These were men in their fifties and sixties.

When you have your bladder removed, your surgeon has to devise an alternative way for you to store and pass urine. This is called a colostomy bag. If bladder cancer goes untreated and advances to Stage 4, then the risk of bladder and prostate removal is very high. This can often result in an inability to have an erection. See how easy it is to let health conditions progress needlessly, making the outcome much worse by your own negligence? That's often what happens when you procrastinate about your health.

Without question, erectile dysfunction is an important area for men, so here's where you need to write a note to self. Just dictate into your smartphone. When you feel symptoms changing in your urination, don't ignore them. Simple enough? One of my best friends called me recently and described classic urinating symptoms that should be looked into, just in case, as a precaution. Right away, after I said he might need to go see a urologist, he objected, "Well, wait a minute. We don't need to go sounding an alarm!" Men, you don't even need a referral to go to a urologist, and this specialist can educate you about what to look for as you age. The field of urology is fascinating, and especially relevant to you. It's like dentistry. If you stay on top of it, you won't dread going.

Men Are from Mars, Women Are from Venus

Have you ever noticed a tendency you have to want to withdraw to a place of solitude when dealing with problems? Or if you just need to get away from the stress? Is this your default method for solving problems? Part of the reason is that we men are by nature happy solving problems, but we like to do it on our own. We'll even gladly solve a problem when no one has asked us to! So, when we're able to withdraw to our man cave and solve a big problem on our own, we feel whole, complete, useful.

This idea of using a man cave as a metaphor grew from my initial exposure to the term twenty years ago in John Gray's 1994 classic, *Men are from Mars, Women are from Venus*. Gray describes how men under certain stressful circumstances want to retreat to their mental man cave in order to solve a problem, or at least do some processing before finally deciding how to deal with the problem. If you think about it, a man cave can either be a physical place you retreat to (like a den or other special room with all a man's favorite electronic toys and creature comforts). Or it can be the most convenient spot available, for example, your bedroom, or even your truck. Gray details how a stressful situation can conjure up a state of mind, where a man checks out mentally and doesn't want to talk about the situation, or even deal with it at the moment, because he needs to go into his "cave" and do some processing.

Lots of men today gravitate to the idea of having a man cave in a literal sense, assigning a room in their home with the specific purpose of providing an escape. They understand full well the benefits of such a refuge, but I'm sure man caves of today go far beyond what Gray had in mind. Even if a man doesn't have a literal retreat to call his man cave, he might nevertheless relax in a place of solitude or just veg out in his favorite chair with his cell phone, playing a video game for an hour. It is his way of disengaging from the stress and strain of the day, hopefully to emerge feeling better.

Women are more inclined to want to talk about their stressful day because sharing problems is a sign of love and trust, not a burden. We men are often ashamed to admit we are even having problems, thinking we don't want to burden anyone. Rarely does a man's ego allow him to openly share his feelings of stress and overwhelm, especially to another man. We don't want to be viewed as weak. We see it is as a threat to our masculinity. As a result, we often end up stuck in a funk.

Guys, one thing I know we do not want to do is get stuck in the cave, because that's where avoidance and procrastination can creep in. Before you know it, it can take over your life and your health, and then it becomes your new friend. That friend you shouldn't hang around with. But you do, anyway.

Man Cave of Health

Some of the man caves we see today are filled with enough "guy toys" to make the average man envious. Overstuffed chairs, pool tables, big-screen TVs, and a bar are just a few of the amenities you might see in one. And with enough money, you can design them to a man's liking in every aspect, from style of décor to theme.

So what's up with this avoidance of doctors men are notoriously famous for? Have you ever considered the reasons—that is, why so many men do such a stupid thing? Have you ever wondered why *you* do such a stupid thing? Men have stated in many surveys that doctors' offices seem to be geared only towards the liking and tastes of moms with kids, or for women, evidenced by the kinds of magazines on the tables and the decor, for example. Now, of course, I'm not saying décor is a valid excuse for avoiding the doctor, but professionals in the medical field are serious about doing a better job of reaching out to men. So give them points for style if you come across a stylish medical facility or doctor's office.

Doctors and medical groups recognize that men are prone to neglect periodic health checkups, then suffer more serious illnesses down the line—many that are preventable and can even prove fatal. It is typical to blame anything or anyone for your shortcomings, but in the case of your personal health and well-being, it is your responsibility. Many of us fail at assuming that responsibility, which is why, as I spell out in more detail in

Chapter 2, in six out of ten leading diseases that cause death—such as heart disease, cancer, unintentional injuries—we have a far higher percentage than women. With a man's health and well-being, simply being male is a risk factor for premature death! I promise not to bore you with too many statistics, because in all the many lectures, webinars, podcasts, and coaching sessions I've done, nothing puts an audience to sleep faster than a bunch of data. The reason simply being male is a risk factor for premature death is, unless men get to the point of emotional pain, they can't relate. Even listening to your doctor go over your blood panel following a physical and making recommendations, chances are, as long as he says you're not going to die, you're good. News flash: You ARE going to die someday, and your doctor with all his knowledge and information on you doesn't know when. So, I say live well while you're still living.

In Chapter 3—A Man Cave of Health—I talk about one of the most progressive medical facilities in the country and what it's doing to provide world-class health care specifically for men, in such areas as prostate cancer, general urology, and erectile dysfunction. The facility has been transformed into a literal man cave setting, complete with sports memorabilia, leather furnishings, coffee bar, and more. And the men who go to this facility can see multiple specialists on the same day, and even go to a pharmacy if needed, for an all-in-one comprehensive visit. A virtual one-stop shop, or Man Cave of Health!

CHAPTER 2

Is There a Gender Health Gap?

The Gender Health Gap

Renowned psychologist and professor emeritus at Stanford University, Philip Zimbardo has lectured for over fifty years on human behavior among other topics. Professor Zimbardo has some interesting insights about the social construct of gender roles. He says:

> Men have a set of rules for what they should _not_ do, but very few men are available to tell them what they _should_ do in order to be a "man." Millions of absentee fathers are spawning a generation of male offspring that have a flawed view of what it means to be a man.

> I submit it begins with how one lives. Most of us go through phases of self-destructive behavior, a

warped mindset, and a long list of dysfunctions
such as eating disorders, emotional dysfunction,
and depression. Once the health goes, it's a steady
decline for millions of men all over the world.
(emphasis added)

These are difficult words to hear because I've lived without a father—someone who was supposed to be there to teach me what I *should not* do, but more importantly what I *should* do—for most of my life. As I shared with you in Chapter 1, the father I loved wasn't equipped to guide his own life, even if he had survived the ravages of alcoholism and its unforgiving outcome. So, much of my life I had to figure things out on my own, and I made plenty of mistakes. But fortunately I had a strong mother who gave me wise counsel about the poor choices Dad had made and how I should learn from them. It helped that I was the oldest of her three children, because I felt a deep sense of responsibility to step up and try to fill the gap that Dad left. I'm sure my two siblings, Jerry and Judy, view me as a father figure in many ways rather than a brother, even though they regard me as their Big Brother.

They looked up to me for support, guidance, and strength, which is something many older siblings are accustomed to, so it wasn't that much of a stretch. Life is faithful to its promise to bring hardships to everyone from time to time, even if you're rich and powerful. That being the norm, we all get numerous opportunities to fail, get up, then try again. That spirit lives in me, and if it doesn't happen to live in you, it can still be awakened; it's never too late. I'm here to bring an awareness to men that we must each take responsibility for ourselves first, and each other whenever we can.

Good gender roles are extremely important, and they play a part in how men view things like masculinity, personal behavior, and even their perspective on health. In my early years, my closest male role model was my grandfather. My grandfather was older than my father would have been of course, but his senior years provided great wisdom since he'd had a chance to mature and grow from his own past mistakes. I was very fortunate to have his good example set before me, in addition to a select few other men in their roles as teachers, pastors, and friends. Some of my coaches were mentors as well, and they definitely influenced my path toward being a stable, healthy, reliable man.

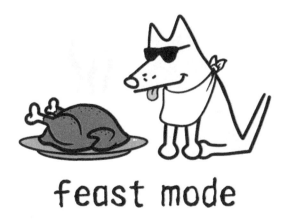

feast mode

For a lot of us men, we've had to figure out life on our own, navigating our way through treacherous waters, using just our instinct at times. In the course of doing so, even though we were told to finish our plate before leaving the dinner table, we may not have made the complete connection between food and health. Leaving the table became the primary motivation for finishing our food! We couldn't care less that eating everything on our plate was good for our health, and of course that depended on what was on your plate.

As boys growing into men, it was normal for us to have a voracious appetite because we were powering through a growth spurt. It didn't matter what we ate; we just needed a lot of it! I can't tell you how many times my mom would catch me in front of the refrigerator with the door wide open, drinking straight out of the milk bottle. It took a while, but eventually, when I started eating out socially and at friend's homes, I got more sophisticated about food and eating. When you hear about a gender health gap, your mind probably conjures up thoughts of some inequity between the two genders at the expense of one. And given that this is a book about men's health, it's safe to assume that I might put forth the idea that men are getting the short end of the stick. You wouldn't be totally wrong, but you might also be a little confused. The fact is, the pendulum swings both ways when you're talking about gender health, and there are plenty of myths and misconceptions to flush out. You might even wonder why gender is important when it comes to health in the first place.

The casual observer might think that health is health, aside from things that are gender specific like breast cancer for women and prostate issues for men. That is an overly simplistic way to view things, but understandable. When it comes to the leading causes of death for humans in general, there are illnesses common to both men and women, but there are mortality rates for cancer for example, that most people would wrongly assume affect women more men. Public perception makes people think that women are stricken with cancer more often than men, but actually more men die from cancer than women. Another mistaken public perception is that men die more often due to heart attacks than women, when in fact the opposite is true.

Regarding cancer, one reason for the misconception is that there's a great deal of attention given to breast-cancer awareness by virtue of the number of marches and other fundraising events in support of it that take place every year. Organizations like the Susan G. Komen Foundation and its annual *Race for the Cure* events do an excellent job. Breast-cancer awareness is a worthy cause to get behind without a doubt. And it is notable to recognize how a pink ribbon has become synonymous with it, thanks to very successful marketing campaigns.

Since the establishment of their "A Crucial Catch" campaign in 2009, the National Football League (NFL) used October as the designated month to promote awareness of breast cancer, and to raise millions of dollars for research and treatment on behalf of the American Cancer Society (ACS). By dressing up the playing field, sidelines, and players in pink gear during certain games in the regular season, they've shown the nation that the NFL is a major player in the fight.

But by 2018 that quietly morphed into a new campaign, which shifted its focus to a broader cancer-awareness effort. The teams and players can still choose breast cancer as their cause, but they can also choose another screenable, detectable cancer such as prostate, colorectal, or whatever a player or coach has a personal tie to. The NFL in a broader sense still uses the pink ribbon logo, but now adds a wider array of colors, including the traditional pink. The vast majority of NFL players in this case stick with their unaltered league gear but actively engage in the promotion of cancer awareness in the community and with league-sponsored media events.

On the other hand, men's health observances like Movember and National Men's Health Month get far less attention. Most people don't even know that the month of June is National Men's Health Month, and the week leading up to Father's Day is National Men's Health Week, started by the US Congress in 1994.

Movember was initiated in 2003 by two mates from Melbourne, Australia, who wanted to bring back the moustache, or "Mo," as a fashion trend. Inspired by a friend's mom who was raising funds for breast-cancer awareness, they decided to use the same fundraising model but in relationship to men's health and prostate cancer. These "Mo Bros" found thirty other guys to grow a Mo during November, and they charged each Bro that grew a moustache $10 for their campaign. As of 2020, the Movember movement has $180 million in total equity, and their global campaign raises funds for a number of male health issues, including mental health/suicide, testicular cancer, and prostate cancer. Last year over 400,000 Mo Bros and Mo Sisters registered to join the global fight. Women raising awareness about breast cancer was the inspiration behind Movember, and women by the tens of thousands volunteer each year to help the cause.

I mentioned heart attacks for men versus women earlier. Early signs of a heart attack are widely and regularly publicized in ads, commercials, and videos. Chest discomfort, arm pain, and shortness of breath are classic symptoms. But they are actually classic symptoms for men who might be having a cardiac episode. For women, their symptoms are not as widely known even to women. Women experience nausea and/or vomiting, jaw pain, and back pain most often when they are having a heart attack. Lack of knowledge of these symptoms in women causes a delay in treatment, sometimes resulting in death. This is a gender-based health gap.

Before we tap into the nuts and bolts of this gender-health gap, let me say for the record that we men come out on the short end of this stick by virtue of the fact that on average our life expectancy is about five years less than women, not to mention the fact that our quality of life leaves much to be desired. In other words, we don't live as well, and we don't live as long. It should also be pointed out that it isn't just because we're male. If anything, it's because we're masculine! A summary of the factors that contribute to this fact are these:

- Men engage in more risky behaviors in recreation and in our occupations

- More men die by suicide than women

- More men die in automobile accidents from drunk driving, speeding, or street racing

- Men tend to avoid doctors more often, ignoring preventive medicine for the most part

- Men abuse alcohol to a greater degree than women

- More men suffer from obesity by not maintaining a healthy weight

- After a certain age more men fail to get sufficient physical exercise

- More men smoke tobacco

As you can readily see, the gender-based health gap is the result of behavior. By common knowledge, everybody knows that most men have a mental block about visiting a doctor. This is a fact we cannot get around; we have to deal with the six-hundred-pound gorilla in the room if we're ever going to come to an understanding about men's health problems. David Thiel, MD, is a urologist at the Mayo Clinic in Jacksonville, Florida. Dr. Thiel says:

> The biggest men's health issue that they should be aware of is that they just don't go to the doctor enough, or they go too late. When you look at men and their relationship with physicians, most don't go until something is wrong. The focus for Men's Health Month is to get men to actually do preventive care, to go to the physician. When men do come in, they're often focused on prostate cancer. However, it's important that most men realize that heart attack, stroke, diabetes, or hypertension are much more prevalent in the population than prostate cancer is. Our biggest issue with men is we know they tend to delay going to a physician unless something's wrong. Women do a much better job of annual or every other year surveillance for things such as cervical cancer, breast cancer and so on.

Dr. Thiel in his statement reveals what so my physicians across the country have known for so long, that the reason for men's health disparities is their own negligence. And it's only getting worse. It's as though men just want to hide in a cave and not come out unless it's absolutely necessary. Were it not for the women in so many men's lives, the mortality rate would be even higher. Avoiding visits to the doctor is only a symptom of the core problem men have.

In my practice, I've come to know that fear is the primary reason men don't go to the doctor. They use a lot of other excuses, but it boils down to that one fact. I've heard with my own ears these fears. "Why should I go to the doctor? All they're going to do is give me bad news!" Talk about a self-fulfilling prophecy. Men hide behind a mask of masculinity and strength, all the while not realizing that observers can see right through their façade. Wives, girlfriends, daughters, and doctors all see it.

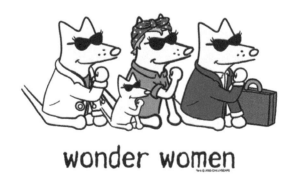

wonder women

Women help close the gap

Four-time *New York Times* bestselling author JJ Virgin is a towering figure in the health and fitness industry. In the much-maligned, gimmicky world of weight loss, JJ Virgin has no peers. She is the premiere voice of scientific reason when it comes to nutrition and wellness (see JJVirgin.com). I was fortunate enough to find *JJ Virgin's Sugar Impact Diet Cookbook* when just starting out as a health coach. I've never been one to read diet books, but I started reading the first few pages, in which she talked about burning fat versus burning sugar, and I was hooked. It was clear to me this was no run-of-the-mill diet cookbook. In fact, just like the title said, it enabled you to reduce the negative impact of sugar on the body through the foods you eat. As a chef, I could definitely relate to all the great recipes with the accurate nutrient content, and I've been able to help my own clients by using them.

For years now, I've been a subscriber to JJ's podcast, *Ask the Health Expert*, where she keeps all her subscribers, myself included, up to date on the latest nutrition tips and information. It enables me to provide expert advice to my clients on a number of important health issues directly. One particular podcast stands out in my mind because she made a reference to herself as the CEO of Health in her home. I identified with that statement immediately because I saw my female clients through that same lens. JJ said that it was a trait so innate in her she would look after the health needs of her husband, her two teenage boys, and even her ex-husband! Kudos to all the women who might be reading this right now if you are the CEO of Health in your home. But shame on you men that require that. You should be the captain of your own ship!

I've had men tell me unequivocally that they wouldn't be alive if it weren't for their wives looking after them. You're blessed if you have a wife who is that nurturing; for most women, it's in their DNA. I know that's the case for my wife, but she also knows that I look after myself primarily. I've been in a few situations where I could not care for myself, and she had my back all the way. I thank God for that and for her. But, guys, we are the ones who should be responsible for the regular maintenance of our own health. That's what a real man does!

Of Mice and Women

Mice have been crucial to the advancement of scientific research and pharmaceuticals. Particularly male mice. They've contributed so much to so many fields that there's even a monument dedicated to laboratory mice on the grounds of the Institute for Cytology and Genetics outside Novosibirsk, Russia. The statue depicts a group of mice (species: Mus musculus) knitting a DNA strand as if it were a sweater. Animal rights advocates, without a doubt, don't like the fact that mice have been and will continue to be used for drug testing and research. But the upside is that the sacrifices of lab mice are responsible for saving millions upon millions of human lives.

There is also a downside, as you might have guessed. Female lab mice have a more complicated hormonal cycle, compared to males. Consequently, scientists prefer using male mice; that way, they can obtain more consistent results. In an article that first appeared in Spectrum News, science journalist Brooke Borel explained how ignoring the differences between male and female lab mice can be very problematic when drugs are approved for human consumption.

Borel described the likelihood that there might be different outcomes based on gender. "A year ago," she stated, "the National Institutes of Health (NIH) rolled out the first phase of a new mandate that requires researchers funded via NIH grants, to either include plans for how they will use animals of both sexes or explain why they will work with only one. The hope is that by studying both males and females, scientists will gain better insights into sex differences ranging from behavior to brain anatomy to drug metabolism." In conclusion, Borel quoted Annaliese Beery, a neuroscientist at Smith College in Northampton, Massachusetts, who said, "The underlying assumption is that if you study males, that's enough and you can extrapolate to everyone else from there. We've seen many examples where that assumption clearly doesn't hold, where there are really important biological sex differences."

Historically, gender was not looked at as a major factor in health, even when scientists thought women due to their hormonal cycle were too variable to use in studies. In addition, there were concerns that pregnant women or their babies might be harmed by experimental treatments, so in 1977 the FDA asserted in a report that women of childbearing potential be excluded from the earliest dose-ranging studies.

Following that 1977 report, except for reproduction studies, most biomedical researchers were reticent to include women. The thought was, it would be easier and more cost-effective to conduct experiments on the male species of mice and on men, generalize the data, then extrapolate to everyone else, notwithstanding the biological differences. As Borel made clear in her article, this assumption did not hold up to scrutiny. Take as a case in point problems infamously revealed with the insomnia drug zolpidem, marketed as Ambien and approved by the FDA in 1992. For years, women complained about experiencing lingering impairment from Ambien—long after it should have been metabolized in their body. Compared to men, women's metabolism is much slower, so the drug remained in their bloodstream twice as long.

It took twenty-one years after the FDA approved the drug for the producers of Ambien to address the dosing problem by cutting the dosage in half in 2013. In 1986, the NIH finally acknowledged that gender does matter by issuing a report stipulating that both sexes should be included in clinical research. In 1993, they backed that report up by requiring that all NIH-funded researchers include more women in their clinical trials.

Today, there have been a number of studies to determine the level of bias toward males in clinical research. Because of the NIH requirement for funding, more than half of the clinical trial participants are now women. However, in preclinical research, the bias towards male laboratory mice is pretty solid at a 5-to-1 ratio at least in the neuroscience category. This shows that we've still got a long way to go. But thanks to the women's health movement that emerged from the 1960s women's equality movement, its political force is alive and well.

As of this writing, I've reached the end of my immunotherapy treatment for bladder cancer. I have a great urologist in Dr. Amit Gupta. He is a very caring physician with a bedside manner that is informative and reassuring. As a result, I have a great deal of confidence in him. Dr. Gupta did all the heavy lifting with my treatment, starting with a minimally invasive surgery and follow-up visits to keep me informed of my prognosis. After my initial surgery, I was relieved to learn I would not need intravenous chemotherapy or radiation. So the immunotherapy I underwent on a weekly basis at a urology clinic has enabled my body to fight off and kill the remaining cancer cells.

It became easy for me to be very comfortable with my weekly treatments, thanks to Dr. Gupta's support staff, who treated me and my wife like family. The nursing staff is professional and competent, and the vast majority of them are women, which struck me as odd for some reason in the beginning. But it actually made more sense once I got engaged with my treatment. Don't get me wrong, Dr. Gupta is extremely skilled in his profession. In fact he is recognized nationally for his competency, and for making Cedars-Sinai Los Angeles one of the leading bladder-cancer treatment centers in the country.

When it came to the weekly immunotherapy treatments, I much preferred that a woman was taking care of me. There's nothing even remotely sexual about the treatments, so don't get that twisted. It's just that the female nurses who have the task of inserting a catheter into my bladder through my penis to deliver medication are much more sensitive and nurturing. That's just my opinion, and I have it on good authority and experience.

Just to give you a little background, the most pain I experienced through my entire treatment came at the hands of the chief resident male physician. My catheter had been removed by my nurse in order to give me an opportunity to urinate on my own before I went home. Unfortunately, I wasn't able to, so he had to reinsert my catheter. This meant I would have to go home with a catheter attached to a portable plastic bag I would carry around with me. My nurses reassured me that having a catheter with me for just a week wouldn't be that bad, and that I'd get to go home once the doctor reinserted that dreaded catheter.

I had to wait for almost two hours for him to arrive, all the while I was pretty anxious to be discharged after twelve long hours in the hospital. I had a sense of relief when he arrived, and he told me he'd have me out of there in no time. That part was true, it didn't take very long. But I had no idea of the excruciating pain I was about to go through. To be fair, it was only a few hours after my surgery, and there was still inflammation, but yeah! In my twelve-immunotherapy sessions, I hardly flinched during the insertion, which means I was in good hands. I understood why some of the men when they checked in were asking if their usual nurse was there that day. They didn't want to trust their body to a different nurse, even though I assume each nurse was every bit as competent as the next.

At the beginning of my health coaching career the majority of my clients were women, and the majority of our conversations during our coaching sessions focused on their spouses. We either discussed what great partners they were in supporting their health goals, or how their spouses needed to join them to regain their health. As time went on, I acquired a most unusual client. Unusual in many ways. Most notably, he was a man: Jim Forte.

Jim has an amazing story. We met at church at a Wednesday morning men's group, where we soon discovered we had something in common. An interest in diabetes. Jim was seventy-seven years young and had been dealing with Type 2 diabetes for nearly fifty years! By then, I was a certified diabetes educator, so I was very interested in knowing more about his condition. Because I had lost my mother to diabetes, it ended up being a motivation for my approach to coaching people with the disease. So, talking with Jim, I became interested in whether I might be able to help him with his condition. Jim sat down with me for an interview about how he came to be diagnosed with diabetes and had been so successful in managing it for decades. Here is a transcription from part of that interview, with only light editing for clarity or length:

Jim Forte Interview

LaRue: *How did you first discover that you had diabetes, Jim?*

Jim: *I was experiencing frequent urination, so I told a buddy of mine who was a pharmacist that I was going through this, and he told me, "Man, it sounds like you've got sugar diabetes." So I went to my doctor and checked it out, and sure enough I was diagnosed with Type 2 sugar diabetes. I couldn't believe it! I was scared. People that had it were dying like flies; it was like polio. I remember it like yesterday. My heart dropped to my knees. It was devastating.*

But because of my faith in God, I decided to look into it to see what I could do to live as long as I could because I didn't think I'd live to thirty. I have a theory about how

I believe it occurred. Before I joined the police force, one of my three jobs was working eight hours a day as a carpenter. Before work, my coworkers and I would stop and get breakfast. We'd eat a big stack of pancakes and syrup and all the rest, and then head off to work. Working hard in the sun for eight hours every day, it was easy to burn off all those carbs and glucose. But after just three months of riding around in a police car all day, the inactivity caught up with me. It was shocking, I mean it was just devastating.

I'd been married for ten years with three kids. Then suddenly I didn't think I'd be around, but thanks be to God, I [decided to do] everything I needed to survive, and I started running five miles every day and doing 200 to 300 pushups every day. That helped me keep my blood sugar down. Nobody knew that I had been diagnosed with diabetes just three months after joining the police force, and they never found out. I made sure I was tops in my class in every physical category, because having to use a needle to inject insulin was not an option. On Culver City's fiftieth birthday, I had become the first black man to ever become a police officer, and I didn't want to give them any reason to fire me. I did all this before becoming the first black man to join the Culver City Fire Department!

LaRue: *So you just learned how to manage the diabetes naturally?*

Jim: Absolutely.

Jim is a remnant of a period when families were larger, and it was understood that the mother ideally would be the housewife, caring for the children while the dad worked outside the home. It was a simpler time, and a household was able to live off of one salary in many cases. Jim embraced the role exemplified to him by his father. He accepted unquestioned the fact that he would be the breadwinner, providing financially for his family. Meanwhile, his wife Jobie took pride in creating a stable home environment.

In certain parts of the country black families were becoming more upwardly mobile through employment opportunities. They embraced in the 1950s and 1960s this opportunity to join the middle class. Although racism was still prevalent in American society, through government legislation and a changing national conscience, our racist past was slowly loosening its grip across the country, and Jim's self-determination and work ethic overshadowed the misguided mindset of some of his fellow citizens.

Imagine if Jim had given up on his personal life goals without even trying, because of his race. He would not have accomplished anything close to what he did. Unlike today, where we as a nation have made astounding progress from our dark past,

Jim's health challenges in face of real racism make him a hero in my book.

Yet the modern feminist movement casts dispersions on the fact that men like Jim were able to make enormous sacrifices on behalf of their families because they had a supportive wife at home. Without them, families like Jim's would not have had such a successful life.

There are millions of men of Jim's generation in which both men and women, in their own way, made their own sacrifices for the benefit of the family. It takes a team to do this, which is why men are just as vital to society as women. Both are vital and important for the sustaining of society.

You could draw the same parallel in terms of his health. Jim faced a situation he didn't expect, Type 2 diabetes. He had two choices. Face his fears, and engage in the fight of his life or submit to his fears and give up on himself. He chose the former, "like a man," in the true embodiment of masculinity. We need more men like Jim Forte, who take innate masculine capabilities like *courage in the face of adversity* or *a determined competition against one's own will* to succeed in doing difficult things. The same abilities athletes rely on in sporting competitions can be summoned to do such noble "Olympic level" feats as defeat a disease like Type 2 diabetes.

Professor Zimbardo goes on to say: So the old traditional roles no longer fit. The old roles were to either be a warrior (soldier) or breadwinner. What's interesting now is that most societies are in transition. As women excel and are doing better and better, there's a whole set of new gender roles that we need to discuss and put into action. The younger generation of women are the legacy of women's liberation from the 70's and 80's, and they create a new problem for boys because girls are doing better and better, while boys are doing worse. Boys are opting out of a confusing world.

Professor Zimbardo believes that boys today are trapped in a hedonistic world, addicted to the instant gratification of gaming and pornography. And they are more likely to be living with their parents, not even helping out with chores or bills. Also, feeling entitled to do nothing. With this self-indulgent mindset, it is easy to see what the future will offer in terms of creating reliable men, ready for the responsibility of marriage and family. Time is running out. I suggest we get busy on ourselves so that we can raise up a useful, functioning next generation.

What's interesting now is that most societies are in transition. As women excel and are doing better and better, there's a whole set of new gender roles that we need to discuss and put into action. The younger generation of women are the legacy of women's liberation from the 70's and 80's, and they create a new problem for boys because girls are doing better and better, while boys are doing worse. Boys are opting out of a confusing world.

What I want to encourage in you is to take the same mindset that a Jim Forte has and apply it to your health. Enter that positive space. Become the hero that your family looks up to you to be, instead of failing at it so often. Our families look to us for encouragement. Inspiration. Too often we let them down. Wearing a mask of false bravado is not masculinity. Most often, people see through it anyway. Facing our fears and moving toward them is what makes you a man, not putting up a false front. Behavior is key to maintaining a state of well-being physically and spirituality that shows your true strength as a man. Take the example of Jim Forte, and create in your mind a "why" for being the best version of yourself you can be.

The Cost of Hiding Emotions

There's a hidden cost to men hiding their emotions. When men struggle with their feelings, it's likely that other men are not available to share with, because they are too busy acting like the typical male, who denies his feelings while pushing other men away to deal with their own feelings. This is the trigger point for dysfunction, which results in men crippled by their behavior.

Men going through these challenges become depressed, turning to alcohol and other drugs to mask their depression. Depression can deepen to where suicide seems to be the best and only escape from the pain. This cycle of behavior is why organizations like Movember are so necessary, as they encourage men to help each other deal with the emotional and even physical challenges they face. Men are not normally inclined to help each other, because we like to go into our cave. But attitudes are changing out of necessity, in an effort to keep up with the times. It would behoove us to take a clue from women in our lives—how they nurture one another in times of need. We can set a better example for younger men, who are struggling more than any generation in history.

Young men, especially, are trapped in this present hedonistic mode where the primary goal of a significant portion is to experience pleasure and avoid pain. But we know that this is not sustainable because even if you bury your head in the sand, the pain is coming. Our society cannot survive if our men and our young men don't become future oriented. And it starts with us. The sad statistic is that more than 40 percent of young boys are growing up without fathers, so they need strong male guidance in order to mature into useful adults. Even if they have a father physically present, some boy's fathers are psychologically absent. So it's clear to see that we are in desperate need of healthy, engaged men present in society. All these indicators point to why men are declining in physical and emotional health, which contributes to the ever-widening gender health gap.

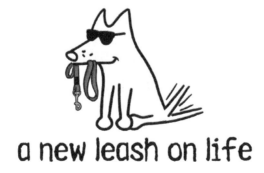

a new leash on life

CHAPTER 3

A New Leash on Life

In 1976 I was forced to leave college at the beginning of my senior year because I had to rescue my mom from an abusive situation with my stepfather in San Diego. There came a time for me in mid-career where the stars were aligned perfectly for me to go back to school and complete my bachelor's degree that I started working toward some forty years prior! It was one of the best decisions I ever made. The fact that I attended a Christian university to complete my degree turned out to be a benefit. It made me look deeper within myself for a career that would utilize a great deal more of my talents and skill set. After I earned a B.S. in Organizational Leadership from Biola University, everything I did from that point on was in preparation for my life's most meaningful work, beginning initially as a chef and culminating with my work in health coaching. By that time I already had the requisite skills to enter the culinary world. I just needed to get some professional experience to back up what I was already prepared to do.

The program took about two years, and when it came time to graduate, I was assigned to a career-guidance counselor. This pivotal moment changed my direction forever. My career counselor recommended that I take the Meyers-Briggs Type Indicator®, a personality test, to best determine what careers suited not only my skill set, but also my aptitude and keen interests. I was starting a new chapter, so my past work experience didn't point me towards what I wanted to do next. The test results were surprising! They revealed that at that point in my life, at fifty-five years of age, the most suitable careers for me centered on three job classifications: teacher, foodservice director, and culinary chef!

The amazing thing is that in the course of five years after receiving my degree, I became all three! Becoming a chef in mid-career was a risky endeavor. I had enjoyed in the past working for major entertainment companies, such as the William Morris Agency, Paramount Pictures, MCA Records, and I even did a stint with the great Quincy Jones at his record company, Qwest Records. Now, after having established myself for twenty-plus years as a high-level executive assistant, it was time to take my street cred into a new environment with unknown challenges, to see if I had what it takes to make the grade.

I started out as a chef working in the assisted-living industry, because I had a great liking and respect for the elderly, and the passion for that work made the job very satisfying. Within a year I showed such a strong acumen for that industry that I left my role as a chef and became a foodservice director at a very high-end assisted-living facility. This was my trial by fire!

Although I ran a major kitchen, my chefs were very accomplished, so they didn't need my expertise in the kitchen. My residents were paying an exorbitant amount of money for luxury accommodations, so they deserved much of my time. But the administrative demands stretched me way too thin. I ended up feeling like a kitchen-based administrator—70 percent of my job was administrative—and it reminded me too much of my many years in the entertainment business. So I made a slight course correction.

I preferred staying in the kitchen, continuing to get hands-on experience in different styles of cuisine, so I ventured into fine dining, which suited me just right. As it turns out, staying in the kitchen, getting hands-on experience with food, broadened my culinary knowledge and expertise beyond my wildest expectations.

I became expert in several cooking styles and could ply my craft in fine dining, catering, and corporate dining. All this by turning my innate abilities in cooking into a career that rewards a strong work ethic, confidence in your skills, and teachability. Good teachers are often very capable learners. I became very adept at learning because I had no fear, believing in my ability to accomplish anything I set out to do. Going back to college at age fifty-five proved to me that I could do anything I desired to do.

SpaceX Launched My Health-Coaching Career

The one thing I can say that launched my career as a chef-turned-health-coach was opening a restaurant for Elon Musk in his SpaceX rocket factory in Hawthorne, California. I signed my employment contract on my sixtieth birthday to become part of the opening team of a brand new, state-of-the-art restaurant and main kitchen. Construction had already begun on the facility when I joined SpaceX, but it took a full six months before we had a functioning restaurant able to feed 5,000 employees per day.

It was during the construction phase of the restaurant that I had my first encounter with Elon, on a day he was giving his now-divorced, *soon to be wife again* Talulah a tour of the main dining room. I was on a break and the couple was trolling the kitchen, looking for someone to prepare them a Valentine's Day lunch. Since I was the only one in sight wearing a chef coat, Elon approached me and asked if there was any food to be had. I introduced myself, then told him I would be able to prepare something for them in very short order.

We were basically a test kitchen at that point, ordering whatever foods we wanted to prepare, as our task every day was to develop new recipes and execute dishes to consider for our menu. I had just finished cooking a delicious batch of braised lamb shanks, so their timing was perfect. I cut my lunch break short and went to work preparing a couple of side dishes to go with the lamb. And just as

I finished plating the meals, the sous chef walked into the kitchen and asked me who the beautiful dish was for. "It's for The Man, and his date!" I replied. The *sous chef* had a stunned look on his face, probably because it would be the first meal that Elon would get to enjoy out of our main kitchen, and he didn't prepare it!

He complimented me on doing such an outstanding job, but asked why I didn't track him down before I did it. I explained that they didn't seem to be in the mood to wait around to eat, so I just took care of it. So, with that explanation he loaded up a serving tray with the plates and some white linens and cutlery, and off he went to deliver Elon's lunch with a very proud look on his face. He returned minutes later to say that it delighted Elon and Talulah to see their sumptuous lamb shank lunch prepared and delivered in record time.

Later I received word from the *sous chef* that Elon loved the lamb shanks, and that no one was to touch the rest of them, as it was one of Elon's favorite foods in life! He ordered the same lamb shank entrée every day after that, until they were all gone! A couple of times I saw the dishes come back from Elon's lunch, where the lamb shank and the starchy foods were the only things eaten, and the vegetables were untouched. That was my first red flag about the dining habits at SpaceX. As a side note, the second time around for Elon and Talulah wasn't a charm, as they remarried only to divorce again a few years later, but at least my lamb shanks were a Valentine's Day hit!

Over budget and behind schedule, construction on the Launch Pad (as we called it) was completed in a few months, and the countdown to officially open for meal service for the employees began. Getting our meal service up and running was the hardest work I'll ever hope to do in life, but after a couple of months we became a well-oiled machine. The SpaceX rocket factory was literally a city within a massive building. The enormous size and scope of the SpaceX complex was a microcosm of society housed under one roof. There was literally a three-story structure within the building, which featured sleeping quarters, offices, and multipurpose meeting space. People from all walks of life and job descriptions spent most of their lives inside this enormous, climate-controlled work environment, and nearly every person within this mini-society relied on our foodservice operation for all their meals.

Elon subsidized all employee meals, so before long the employees were able to have breakfast, lunch, and dinner while at work. Meals cost a mere five dollars, plus Elon paid thousands of dollars for other perks, like free barista coffee, frozen yogurt, chips, fruit, bottled water, and a wide variety of fountain beverages. It did not take long for this massive food distribution program to give me a pretty accurate profile of the eating habits of most of the employees, which would give me some invaluable insights into human behavior.

The primary facility was the central kitchen, an exhibition-style kitchen which was state-of-the-art in every respect. I've worked in plenty of exhibition kitchens before, and it's a lot like you're on stage every moment of your shift. Initially there was a lot of competition to work on the front line. We called it "the Show" because you were the center of attention. But I wanted no part of that. Working the grill or being on the front line might look glamorous and cool, but you soon find out the job can wear you down like no other because the work pace is brutal. Such is the life in a production kitchen, where you're required to produce high volumes of food under pressure in an environment that is bustling, noisy, and hot.

When we opened for business, the executive chef put me on the serving line because he wanted a more experienced chef to represent the face of the crew, rather than a deer staring at headlights. The job called for maturity, professionalism, and experience, as we wanted to present this new experiment as a solid operation. So it was a great opportunity to set a good example for others to follow, as well as to show my leadership abilities under pressure. There were some growing pains to be sure, but in a few months we got things under control, and the department established itself as a professional food service entity that was a staple operation.

Because of my growing interest in whole-food nutrition, I jumped at the opportunity to manage the enormous salad bar, which was an asteroid of fresh salad fare, composed salads, whole fruit, and dressings that had to be maintained and restocked throughout the day. Since I was the chef in charge of that area, I got to know a lot about people's interest in healthy eating. Hundreds of individuals every day thrived on the salad bar and its wide variety of fresh food, while others steered clear of it, opting for the usual burgers, sandwiches, and breakfast fare they were more accustomed to. What stood out to me was that most people, especially the men, did not know what a balanced diet was. It was at this point that I began to identify myself as a healthy food advocate, and I welcomed the challenge.

During my tenure at SpaceX, I enrolled in the Institute for Integrative Nutrition, the world's largest nutrition school, headquartered in New York City. It is the longest-running online institution dedicated to the teaching of nutrition concepts for health coaches, as well as business training to assist its graduates in setting up their health coaching practice. The curriculum was intensive and lasted two years, during which time I continued to work ten to twelve-hour shifts, six days a week. Between my studies and what I viewed as my very own food-and-nutrition lab at SpaceX, I was never lacking in examples of both good and bad eating habits. Many SpaceX employees showed a keen interest in learning as much as they could from me about a healthy diet and lifestyle, so you could say I began my health coaching internship in the rocket factory.

Unsurprisingly, there were far more examples of bad eating habits to observe, and I saw the results of those poor dietary and lifestyle choices evidenced by the ever-increasing size of many of the customers we served day in and day out. There were two people in particular, a man and a woman, whom I watched over a four-year span gain at least a hundred pounds each! That sounds incredible, but when you consider how easy it was to overindulge in a variety of unhealthy foods without being encouraged to make better choices, it was inevitable. They wore the same type of clothes and shoes every day, so it was clear they were literally growing out of them.

The SpaceX campus was massive, covering several city blocks. We eventually had to open up satellite food outlets at the most populated worksites. One of my various assignments was an offsite machine shop blocks away from the man campus, where I developed some very interesting relationships with pretty sizable crews of the guys (and some girls!) who worked there, and we talked a lot about diet and nutrition. They became keenly interested in my ongoing studies in nutrition, so they always came with questions about what they should order, helpful weight-loss advice and nutrition tips, and what to do about certain health conditions they were experiencing.

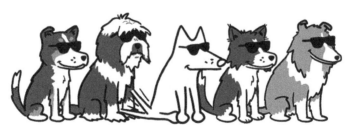

this is your wake up collie

Several individuals diagnosed with Type 2 diabetes were struggling with understanding what comprised a low-glycemic diet, while others were trying to get their weight under control. Those under the care of a doctor complained that at no time did they receive any advice about diet and nutrition as it related to their diabetes, only prescriptions for either Metformin or insulin to control their elevated blood sugar. When I explained that diabetes was a lifestyle disease, they felt the doctors they were seeing cared only about pushing drugs on them for profit, and had no concern for them to ever get better. Some of the crew came seeking advice on how to take knowledge home to their loved ones who desperately needed intervention to help deal with the debilitating conditions of Type 2 diabetes. Since I had expertise in addressing diabetes self-management issues, I ended up getting a number of clients simply by giving away knowledge for free. I had earned their trust because they were starting to see results in weight loss and a reduction in medication.

I took a special interest in anyone who approached me with questions about diabetes, because my mom died years before due to complications from undiagnosed diabetes. In fact, I had to sue my mom's doctors just to find out why she was sent home following an examination and blood tests, only to suffer a diabetic stroke the next day. Two days after visiting her doctor, my mom died from a diagnosable condition from a treatable disease. As a result, I became well versed in diabetes and how pervasive it is in our country and the world. Clearly, she didn't have to die, so it became my mission to do my best to prevent anyone I can from suffering the same fate as she.

Several employees I served had been diabetic for several years, but they did not know how critical a role proper diet and exercise played. The primary reason is that we do not train doctors to look at diabetes as a lifestyle disease that is preventable, and sometimes reversible. We train most doctors to treat the symptoms of the disease with medication, so the disease continues to progress because they ignore the root cause which is insulin resistance.

I began dispensing useful information—to a few people at first, but as my reputation grew, so did my audience. People would line up for their meal, and the guys I was coaching would come to my window and say, "Just serve me what you think I should eat!" It's surprising how quickly I got into the heads of people seeking my advice. They would tell me they could hear my voice in their head when they were eating at home, and especially at a restaurant. And the worst part of all is that none of the information I was giving them had they heard from their doctors, only what medicines to take.

Manny was a test technician who came to my food trailer every day for breakfast and lunch. All the men he hung out with knew him for both his poor eating habits and that he was diabetic. The guys he took breaks with had given up on trying to encourage him not to eat bad foods that would raise his blood-sugar levels, and they told him often to at least have some vegetables or a salad with his meal. Manny always turned down the vegetable sides I would offer with his plate, and he liked to double up on a starch, like rice or potatoes instead.

One day Manny was standing in line with a few of his buddies who liked to refer to me as the health guy. We were serving fajitas for lunch, and he wanted me to pick out as much of the peppers and onions as possible, and add more meat. He also requested rice and beans and extra tortillas. "Damn dude, you're gonna kill yourself," blurted out his friend. That's how I learned everyone knew he was diabetic. His friend called him out and said he should listen to what I had to say about diabetes. I let him know my background, and that I was interested in helping him with his diabetes if he wanted me to.

Years earlier when he was diagnosed, all he understood about his condition was that he could take Metformin (a common drug for diabetics) twice a day, to keep his blood sugar under control. His doctor may or may not have told him about diet and exercise, but all he heard was that you could take the pills, and everything would be under control. In all honesty, only a small percentage of doctors take the self-management approach to treating diabetes, but immediately put their patients on a medication that only deals with the symptoms. Based on Manny's reaction, I assumed that most of what I shared with him was news to him.

What Manny did not know was that when the Metformin was no longer effective in keeping his blood sugar in check, he would have to transition to taking insulin shots. He rarely tested his blood sugar, but complained about increased symptoms. I met with him after work one day and gave him a thorough briefing on how diabetes affects the body, and that it could lead to many other conditions, including heart disease and stroke, which got his attention. It has been my practice to take people I coach to their pain point as quickly as possible, so that they understand they have a serious problem. I let them know the bad news of what will happen if they ignore my advice about diabetes self-management, and I go into great detail. I often share the story about my mom's situation, and why I'm so passionate about the subject. Eventually, I give them the good news that a qualified diabetes educator, like myself, is trained to help them make that change if they so desire. Like most people, Manny had a hard time believing that eating what he wants every day was jeopardizing his health.

He never ate vegetables because he just didn't like them. He hadn't tried very many, but those he tried, he didn't like ever since childhood. It was as though eating a vegetable was not very masculine to him. Like hundreds of men I've spoken to about this, his view was that men work hard, play hard, so they need food for strength and endurance, like steak or chicken, the best sources of protein for a man. In his mind, eating salads was a "girl thing." Notice how easily views of masculinity creep in relating to food and eating habits?

Many a man has declared at the dinner table to just pass the steak, pass the mashed potatoes and gravy, but keep that rabbit food away from me! Eating as though passing on vegetables is a badge of honor for men gets reinforced from an early stage, when a man's body is developing as a teenager. Lots of men declare themselves to be strict carnivores, but they really don't know what they are saying. My cat is a carnivore! Humans are omnivores, which means we eat both meat and plants. This faulty logic can over time turn into an eating disorder and is especially misleading if a man's weight seems to be under control. Age plays a factor in this because as the male body changes from being able to handle this kind of diet regimen, he can end up being TOFI (thin outside, fat inside).

That happened to me! Here I was, a brand-new, certified health coach, signing up for a gym membership just to help maintain my good health. When my trainer took my measurements of body fat, weight, height, etc., she chuckled and said, "You're what we call skinny fat!" Whaaat! Much to my surprise, body mass index (BMI) was in the high twenties and that is not good. I had convinced myself that I was the picture of health because I looked relatively fit in my clothes. I had to get over myself and realize I'd been reading my own press clippings. When my trainer crunched the numbers, it turned out I needed to follow some of my own advice and become more conscious of my state of health, regardless of what I thought. The visceral fat stored deep in my body impacting my organs was a definite health risk that I needed to address.

Since we're talking about food, as the old saying goes, "Someday your chickens will come home to roost!" In a more modern translation, your body will one day collect on the debt you owe! As I've stated before, but it bears repeating, years of unhealthy eating and living can take its toll on your body, which will either begin the decline of your *healthspan,* or you can respond by turning back the clock, opting for an alternative lifestyle that extends it to last about as long as your lifespan. The way to do that is to give it the fuel that it needs instead of the sugar and the carbohydrates it doesn't need. Food is fuel! When you do that, you won't have to spend the latter part of your life suffering from a lifetime of poor eating and physical inactivity.

Men, we have a lot of common concerns and conditions, and though we've been maligned by the current radical feminist revolution, we <u>are</u> essential; we <u>are</u> needed, and we <u>are</u> a valuable part of our society and culture. As men, we need to reclaim our right to relevance in an ever-changing culture that is at times anti-male. We're led to believe that our inclination to be aggressive and competitive is toxic and must be suppressed; we must resist that and not become passive. Some male behavior has been toxic, that is true. But not all masculine behavior is toxic behavior, and we have the power to change and redefine our own image. The answer to toxic masculinity is not no masculinity; it's better masculinity, and I say that it is very masculine to be more intentionally conscious about our health.

My years at SpaceX opened my eyes to how our society can get offtrack in terms of health, and based on my observation, the reversal starts with making better lifestyle and behavior choices, and having better attitudes about health. It was a very interesting four-year experience observing how thousands of people behaved towards food, especially because it was abundant, easily accessible, and they had multiple choices of food of all types, at a minimal cost.

In the next chapter, we'll examine what the medical profession is doing to respond to a growing crisis of men's health. Hospitals and medical centers all over the country are developing creative and effective ways to raise awareness which is only the first step. Only action on our parts will change the narrative. Recognizing that there is a clear gender health gap as discussed in Chapter 2 is not enough. We must come together like a band of brothers to help ourselves and other men and boys overcome this trend. Simply being male is not the health risk. It's the male misperception of "masculine" that is the real health risk!

CHAPTER 4

A Man Cave of Health

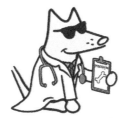

trust me I'm a dogtor

There's a need for an approach to men's health that addresses men's specific concerns such as sexual function, prostate issues, avoidance of heart disease, and maintaining a healthy weight and optimal performance in a way that is responsive, approachable, and thorough.

—Dr. Myles Spar

An increasing number of medical centers and hospitals recognize that declining health in men is a growing problem. Health practitioners are looking for alternative ways to attract men and get them interested in taking better care of their health. It's one thing to acknowledge the seriousness of a problem that needs dealing with, but getting to the root cause is much more complex. Let's dispense with the typical diet-and-exercise routine and get to the primary cause, which is *behavior*. Underlying that concern is a man's mental attitude, or mindset, about health altogether.

There are myriad reasons for the declining state of health of men the world over, especially in the US, but you can never get on-target toward understanding why until you realize that attitude and behavior are the keys to optimal living and longevity. Make it your mantra that healthspan and lifespan go together as one.

If someone were to ask you to define what men's health is, you might be hard pressed to come up with an accurate definition. I'd be happy to give you my definition, but let me begin by stating that it is not simply the absence of disease or other infirmity. The magazine *Men's Health* is the most popular "men's health" title at newsstands, but has a limited scope in terms of health matters men face. The cover features mostly celebrity athletes or actors who are in great shape, and the articles inside are usually fluff pieces. You're also likely to find a workout plan that promises to help you get 6-pack abs in 28 days. Most of the men past the age of forty have likely moved on with life and don't have the time or inclination to obsess over trying to build a head-turning physique. For them, the Dad bod is more their speed!

Men's health, in a nutshell, encompasses physical, mental and social well-being; however, what deems a man to be healthy is the elusive part. In Chapter 2, I spoke about how men continue to comprise most of the major categories of research subjects in scientific studies of diseases that occur in both men and women. In this model, men's health is viewed as anything not related in particular to women's health. Clearly, a somewhat limited view that misses the importance of coming up with medications and treatments specific to men, such as for erectile dysfunction, prostate disease, and low testosterone. These conditions have a disproportionate impact on men's health in relation to heart disease and to death due to lifestyle factors.

Today, integrative health is a relatively new field of medicine that can bring hope to patients, because it is a relationship-centered health-care model that focuses on prevention and health-promoting lifestyle, something that men can benefit from. This patient-centered care model is a game changer. It empowers patients to actively participate in their own health and self-healing as they learn to understand all the factors at work. Men especially benefit from understanding how body, mind, spirit, and community are essential to optimal health. In the field of integrative health for men, *Integrative Men's Health*, by Myles D. Spar, MD, MPH, and George E. Munoz, MD, is a seminal work. In the introduction, Dr. Munoz writes, "In the traditional Western medicine model, men's health as a specific field of recognition and importance has until recently received anemic recognition and marginal attention by most health professionals. Furthermore, a unique field of male health is needed to better understand how to address the needs of men, who present differently than women even when suffering from the same conditions as women."

It seems shocking, but outside of the internet and some select books, there are very few sources of information and care related to men. In an effort to face that challenge, Mount Sinai Health System, New York, launched a first-of-its-kind resource center for men called Man Cave Health. The nonprofit organization Man Cave Health is the namesake of the center, giving its moniker to the urology department chaired by Dr. Ash Tewari. The initial goal of this partnership was to provide educational resources for men regarding prostate health, that treatable, male-specific condition that far too many men know little about. By incorporating the comfort concept of a man cave, Mount Sinai transformed its waiting room into a sports-themed facility, with the intent of appealing to men who appreciate sports and a guy-centered environment. New York being the sports mecca it is, the waiting room is bedecked with sports jerseys and gear autographed by some of the most high-profile players from many of the various professional sports teams that hail from the city.

The urology center is a one-stop shop for treatment of a wide range of male-specific conditions, including prostate health and erectile dysfunction. The waiting room features comfortable leather seating, a 70-inch big-screen television, and a free-coffee bar, besides consultation and health services specific to men only. According to the American Cancer Society, prostate cancer is one of the most common cancers men get, second only to skin cancer, and if caught early is not fatal. Erectile dysfunction (ED) is another condition that men experience at a rate of 10 percent per decade of life: 50 percent of men in their fifties, 60 percent of men in their sixties, etc. In terms of raw numbers, 30 million men in the US, according to the National Institute of Diabetes and Digestive and Kidney Diseases (NIDDK).

Thomas Milana Jr., an advocate for men suffering from prostate cancer, pioneered the Man Cave Health program following his own diagnosis in 2016. He had successful surgery at Mount Sinai performed by Dr. Tewari, who has done over six thousand robotic radical prostatectomies. Dr. Tewari has a passion for getting a message to men, especially as they age. He states, *"I think men don't take care of their health as well [as women]. Men take better care of their cars than their bodies, and that needs to change. Man Cave Health is a fresh way of starting a conversation about issues that men don't enjoy talking about."*

Milana and his organization plan to open many more Man Cave Health centers in hospitals across the country run by their urology departments, that will reach out to men needing prostate-specific antigen (PSA) screenings. For most men, prostate issues and erectile dysfunction are top-of-mind awareness, and the Mount Sinai center understands the sensitivity around these concerns. Once men enter the center, they have access to other screenings in the same day, that can help head off such things as heart attack, stroke, or diabetes, which are much more prevalent in men than prostate cancer or erectile dysfunction.

Several hospitals in the US are taking cues from organizations like Man Cave Health, providing male-specific education, diagnosis, and treatment in a more masculine environment, replete with nontraditional décor, using more corporate or sports themes, instead of the usual clinical setting that is a traditional turnoff to most men.

Millions of men lack a sense of the need to be proactive about their health, and by avoiding regular doctor visits, they make it impossible to engage in any early disease detection. This behavior is increasing the chances of many preventable diseases developing, something far too common for millions of men. And when men underuse the health care available to them and more serious conditions strike, instead of the much lower preventative-care costs, they end up requiring the much more expensive hospital care, thus burdening our nation's already broken and overutilized health-care system. According to recent CDC statistics, chronic disease in the US has a major impact on the nation's economy. Heart disease and stroke take 868,000 American lives every year, which amounts to one-third of the deaths. The economic toll on our health-care system is $214 billion per year, which causes a $138 billion loss in job productivity. I've spoken to many men who just don't expect to live a long life, which is clear by the way they live out their lives. Some call it "going for the gusto," but I call it driving the car until the wheels fall off. I relate quality of life to being motivated to continue living, but it takes a sense of purpose I call contending for your "why." Why should you strive to sustain your health as long as possible? What is so important that you should feed your body and keep your mind focused on living the best life possible? These are questions you may never have considered before, but that beg answering. We will delve into the most obvious reasons later, but for now let's examine the various means by which we can accomplish the goal of living well and long. Come into the man cave of health!

Think of your man cave as a virtual place similar to the one in Mount Sinai Hospital. Imagine it supported by your doctor or medical care team, which can include your family, other loved ones, even close friends. A mixture of key elements can work together for your good, but you have to go after it.

> *"For I know the plans I have for you," declares the LORD. "Plans to prosper you and not to harm you, plans to give you hope and a future."*
> —Jeremiah 29:11

Before the global pandemic of 2020, America was already in a state of declining health, and men led in six out of ten categories for highest mortality. The pandemic only made it more apparent what a good deal of health practitioners have known for years—that America is getting sicker and sicker and that men lead in the majority of major categories. The Centers for Disease Control (CDC) predicted that those at the highest risk for contracting COVID would be seniors of a certain age with preexisting, or underlying, conditions.

Among that high-risk group with preexisting health conditions in the US, men had the highest percentage of hospitalizations and deaths, and ethnic minorities in the lower-income brackets topped that list overall. This glaring disparity in outcomes was disconcerting, but a closer examination of lifestyle choices, diet regimen, and behavior revealed that the primary factor contributing to poor health outcomes—regardless of financial or social status—was personal responsibility. Media and the medical profession pay far too little attention to this, and whenever the subject is brought up in the media, there is pushback from members of those ethnic-minority groups, as well as several media outlets and political figures. The default assumption is that if there is a disparity in health outcomes, the cause must be racism. Men in general minimize their health concerns, often viewing them as a sign of vulnerability. For some, that mindset comes from playing competitive sports. Playing injured is part of sports culture, and having been an athlete in high school and college, playing football, baseball, and track and field, I know that firsthand. The coaches encouraged it, and we wanted to emulate the tough-guy image they were fond of, so we didn't want to ever let them know if we were too hurt to practice. Our innate competitive nature caused us to play through the pain and not disappoint our coaches or our team in our quest to win. Today, organized team sports at the high school, college, and even professional level are much more careful about allowing athletes to continue practicing or playing while injured, because so many have suffered debilitating and even life-threatening aftereffects. And of course there are concerns about lawsuits, ever since a number of student athletes died on the practice field.

This is the mindset that doctors and medical professionals have to deal with in men, which makes their job even more difficult than it already is. As a result, a lot of creative effort by doctors, hospitals, and medical facilities goes into generating interest and concern in men to be proactive about their health. Wives and significant others show more concern for men's health than they themselves do, and as a result have saved many lives.

In our politically correct environment in America, whenever there is a public emphasis towards men and their health, it's likely that some will assume it is at the expense of women. Clearly, that is not the case. Men's health and women's health are both important for the benefit of the country. Families, businesses, and society will win when men embrace optimal health. And when men don't do well, our country doesn't do well.

Start a Men's Health Movement

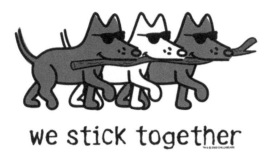

I believe men should start a "bro-ification" of health movement, which means men throughout the country and the world should join forces, nurturing relationships among each other, and even form support groups that bring awareness to the health problems men face. Medical clinics and volunteer organizations would welcome the opportunity to support groups like that.

If you can, identify even one man you can call your "bro," whom you can trust with sensitive personal information. I encourage men everywhere to "man up" to this looming health crisis. It might surprise you how supportive another man might be—which might give both of you the courage to take that first step of getting over the fear you've conjured up in your head. We all do it, and it's always wrong. Are we not men? Aren't we the ones that stare down fear on the battlefield for a noble cause? I can think of nothing more noble than to keep your health in check so that you are ready for whatever battle you might face.

Millions of men have grown up with wrong-minded thinking about what it means to be and act like a man. It is certainly not manly to hide physical pain, for fear of what the doctor might reveal. I call that just plain stupid. Make up any excuse you want, but at some point, you're going to end up having to pay a visit to a doctor. It will be your primary care physician, an emergency room doctor, or the coroner. While you still can make a choice, I urge you to choose now to do the right thing, if only so that you don't become an enormous financial and emotional burden on your entire family.

Consider my man cave of health idea as a virtual realm in your mind focused on strengthening men, like iron sharpening iron. Your doctor can be part of your man cave. Another man or men can occupy a supportive role as well.

The world knows that men do a poor job with their health. To prove the point, we see statistics year after year that remind us that women on average outlive men by five years. And even though that gap is widening since the COVID pandemic, it still seems to be just a number to many men. Men tend to be natural-born leaders, but when we don't embrace that tendency within us to lead in more meaningful ways, we seem to wander through life. If I didn't strive every day to be a responsible, compassionate leader in my home, my wife would take over. Why? Because she can do so if necessary. And she would resent me for letting this happen. Most wives don't want to have to wear the pants. They want us to take the mantle and step up for our families as the men we claim to be.

That's why I look at men's health as something that needs to become goal centered. When we hear talk about BMI or being overweight, or perhaps getting our numbers within some arbitrary reference range, for some of us our eyes glaze over. It doesn't motivate us. But if you have an endgame, such as in the earlier example of coaching your youngest daughter's soccer team, that's a realistically achievable goal. It's more doable to start a conditioning regimen scalable to our need to bond with our child, provided we cherish that relationship enough to do so.

Most of us have conditioned ourselves to be tough, self-reliant breadwinners, but without regard for our own personal health: We engage in high-risk jobs and behaviors; we consume food and drink that acts like poison to our bodies; and we manage stress poorly because we think men can handle the stress naturally. This behavior is toxic to our health and well-being, and much of it falls under the belief that we are acting like men. We are acting like millions of men do, but that's why we are an endangered species!

Men tend to have an interesting dynamic when it comes to their doctor/patient relationship, especially if they prefer a male doctor. They might have intentionally chosen a male based on the belief that men are more competent. But according to a 2014 Rutgers study, men will paradoxically be less open about their symptoms to the male doctor. Researchers Mary S. Himmelstein and Diana T. Sanchez, in "Masculinity Impediments: Internalized Masculinity Contributes to Healthcare Avoidance in Men and

Women," first published Oct. 7, 2014, explained: *"That's because they don't want to show weakness or dependence to another man, including a male doctor."* Ironically, the researchers found, men tend to be more honest about their medical symptoms with female doctors because, Sanchez theorizes, to be honest about vulnerabilities causes them no loss of status with women.

Both men and women were part of the study, and as the Rutgers article by Ken Branson, "The Tougher Men Think They Are, the Less Likely They Are to be Honest Doctors," indicates, it turns out, exaggerated self-reliance can be dangerous to health. "It's worse for men, however," says Himmelstein, co-author of the article originally published in the *Journal of Health Psychology*: "Men have a cultural script that tells them they should be brave, self-reliant and tough. Women don't have that script, so there isn't any cultural message telling them that, to be real women, they should not make too much of illnesses and symptoms."

A fact worth noting is that if a man is in his late thirties to forties and experiences erectile dysfunction, it could be a precursor to certain forms of cardiovascular disease. Some degree of ED might be typical in men of a more advanced age, but for a younger man it could be a sign of trouble. Regular doctor visits increase the likelihood of early detection and treatment of heart disease, reducing the risk of a serious cardiac event down the line. The biggest issues men face is that they just don't go to the doctor often enough, or when they do, it's too late. It's a very good idea to be honest with your doctor, and do your best to establish mutual trust. If that's not possible, look for another doctor—do an interview online, do your homework. That way, you're being your own health advocate.

Once men reach a certain age, usually around fifty, they need to monitor certain conditions that might be early warning signs for health issues peculiar to men. Even when your doctor says your numbers look good, ask her what were your numbers from your last physical and have they increased slightly? You should develop an informed interest in your health by asking your doctor to tell you what your optimal range is and what to do if your numbers venture outside of that range. Blood sugar, blood pressure, and other measures all have optimal ranges that change as you age. Saying your numbers look good doesn't mean anything if they're creeping up gradually and you're not making a comparison.

I speak from personal experience because when I was diagnosed with bladder cancer, every time I went in for my immunotherapy my vitals were checked. Each time the nurse checked my blood pressure reading, it was too high, even though from my annual physical exams, I had no knowledge of even elevated blood pressure. So I contacted my primary-care physician, but he had no openings for several weeks. I asked to be scheduled with the first available doctor, which was less than a week away. He did a thorough blood pressure exam, and we spent about an hour together looking over my health history, assessing what lifestyle and diet habits could be improved.

For years, it turned out, my blood pressure had been elevated past the optimal reference range, and hypertension definitely ran in my family. We decided to put me on medication immediately, while at the same time I would work on improving my sleep habits, getting my weight down, and increasing my exercise regimen so that I could eventually control my blood pressure naturally. My hope is that I can get my numbers into a healthy range without the need for medication. But first things first. I had to get on medication because my blood vessels have been under increased strain already. Hypertension is nothing to play with. It can easily lead to a stroke if you're not monitoring your health in this important area.

Take the condition known as insulin resistance. Insulin resistance progresses over many years and is one reason you experience escalating weight, growing inches around the waist, and a sense of always being hungry. In terms of numbers, a normal blood pressure reading should be close to 120/80. A blood pressure reading of 130/80 is cause for concern.

A fasting blood glucose reading over 100 mg/dl, or fasting triglycerides over 150 mg/dl is also reason to discuss with your doctor ways of bringing those numbers in the normal range without drugs. These are not alarming numbers, but if there has been a gradual increase over a few years, I would say it's time to look at preventative measures before your doctor prescribes medication to bring those numbers into a normal reference range.

I base those reference ranges on averages of a "healthy" group of individuals. But not everyone is typical. Some healthy individuals can have readings outside the normal reference range, while unhealthy people can have readings within the normal reference range. Optimally, you want to look at those numbers as they relate specifically to you, which requires more discussion with your physician, especially if you have a family history of disease that you wish to avoid or at least manage.

Out of approximately two hundred different countries in the world, there are several different health-care systems used among them, with the same goal in mind: to provide adequate health care to all citizens at an affordable price. However, the focus, in most cases, is on pharmaceuticals to treat symptoms of disease rather than on understanding and addressing the underlying cause. Medical schools are not training doctors in nutrition and disease prevention. Instead, in the case, for example, of a nutritional disease like Type 2 diabetes they learn to treat the symptoms with drugs, which won't cure the disease but actually sustains it as the disease progresses. When you treat only the symptoms that have their root cause in lifestyle, the disease continues to worsen, leading to comorbidities. Comorbidities are two or more diseases present simultaneously in the same individual that sometimes relate to the primary disease, such as high blood pressure being a comorbidity of Type 2 diabetes.

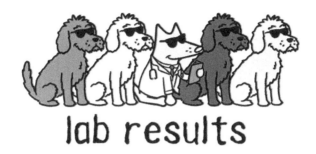

lab results

Once a man reaches the age of fifty, there are several health screenings he should not miss, in addition to certain conditions he should monitor, that can save him a lot of grief later. Under no circumstance should you go through life assuming that you're fine if you haven't been to see a doctor in years. That doesn't mean you're healthy, just that you can't hear the ticking time bomb loud enough. Eventually, things will begin to break down because these bodies of ours have an expiration date, some sooner than others. And just as with an automobile, our warranty can be voided if we don't take care of the regular maintenance. Consider these guidelines:

• Physical Examinations (every year)

• Colonoscopy (every ten years)

- Blood pressure (every year)

- Fasting blood sugar Glucose (every year)

- PSA/Digital Rectal Exam (DRE)

- Cholesterol (every year if overweight)

- Fasting Insulin Test (every year if overweight)

- Dental examination/cleaning" (twice a year)

- Eye examination (Age 50+ every 1-3 years)

CHAPTER 5

New Health Rules for Men

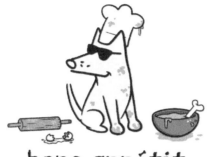

bone appétit

Some of you may remember the Popeyes® Crispy Chicken Sandwich craze that caused mayhem a couple of years ago. That sandwich, a crispy deep-fried chicken breast on a toasted brioche bun with pickles and either mayo or spicy sauce, was the flashpoint for a number of physical altercations, involving knives, guns, fists—and even cars! People lost their minds, and one unfortunate man lost his life.

The YouTube channel *In The Loop* played a video of a determined patron of a Popeye's restaurant drive-in in Los Angeles where a woman in a Mercedes tried to cut in front of other cars. In her futile attempt to squeeze ahead in the line, she got boxed out, trapped between other customers in line and a concrete post. As bystanders looked on, she proceeded to badly scrape the entire side of her car, taking the only exit route the other cars would allow. The videographer recording the incident panned over to a bystander watching the ordeal while enjoying one of the coveted sandwiches herself.

You could hear the inquisitive filmmaker asking her, "Damn, is it *that* worth it?" As the woman was about to devour the last bite of her sandwich, without a word she responded with an earnest nod, "Yes!"

The public demand for this iconic bundle of gastric pleasure food even cost one man in Prince George's County, Maryland, his life. Kevin Tyrell Davis was stabbed to death for methodically taking cuts in a fifteen-minute line of people waiting to order the coveted sandwich. Davis's assailant, who fled the scene, was apprehended by police after ten days on the run. Channel 13 WJZ televised Ricoh McClain being taken into custody, whereupon he was charged with first-degree murder and assault. Over a chicken sandwich! In this demonstration of toxic masculinity, the victim's determination to gain access to an unhealthy fast-food sandwich out of turn proved to be a startling example of something unworthy of the sacrifice.

In another sense, it is striking how radical human behavior can become. When you consume foods low in nutrient density, your body will continue to "crave" the nutrients it is seeking from your diet. It's just like when the engine light comes on in your car's dashboard, alerting you that there's some type of maintenance required. Many of us respond to those cravings, consuming foods that will not satisfy the body's need for glucose from a healthy food source. Our body is a finely tuned metabolic organism, engineered to repair and maintain itself provided we give it the right fuel at the right time. Unless and until you give your body the proper fuel it needs to run optimally, that engine light is going to stay on!

A few years ago, a friend of mine had a hit television show, *Man vs. Food*, on the Travel Channel. Adam Richman starred in this popular show that combined a type of toxic masculinity in the form of aggressive eating disorder, with gluttony which is one of the Seven Deadly Sins. Now here are two behaviors that are particularly harmful to the body for two reasons. Firstly, if you engage in what I call sport eating, your body valiantly tries to deal with the surge of not only large amounts of animal protein and saturated fat, but a boatload of carbs and added sugars as well.

As the show's host, Adam was to visit a popular local eatery some-where in the country each week, prepared to take on the challenge of gobbling up the most iconic, obnoxious item on their menu, usually one of gargantuan size, and he would do it on camera. Adam faced some very daunting eating challenges along the way, but to his credit he met every challenge. However, after four years of competitive eating, he simply lost interest in it. It was rumored that he had suffered health setbacks from the show, which would not surprise me, but more likely Adam Richman felt he had bested his worthy opponent, food, so there was nothing left to prove.

Subjecting your body to this kind of onslaught on a sustained basis can damage your health later in life, and that's what a lot of men do, only to a lesser degree.

Granted, this is an extreme example, but many people find this kind of behavior entertaining, great for shock value but also typical behavior of men. And where does it get you? The host of *Man vs. Food* got paid for his antics, but he also candidly shares in interviews the price he paid afterwards for winning every challenge, especially in the case of things like ghost peppers and chili extracts in the dish.

In real life there are guys that eat this way, and the sad part is they do it for free! What I've come to know in my practice is that people in general, and men in particular, are "present biased" in that they don't worry too much about the damage gluttony might cause to their future health, when a twenty-four-inch Chicago Deep Dish Pizza is staring up at them in the here and now!

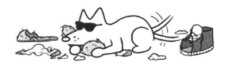

chew the right thing

Most of the chronic diseases men suffer from today are life-style-driven, and thereby avoidable. Some of those preexisting conditions include obesity, heart disease, fatty liver disease, high blood pressure, and Type 2 diabetes, to name a few. And when you consider that unless absolutely necessary, men intentionally avoid going to the doctor, no wonder men lead in nine of the top ten causes of death in the U.S. When we examine what kinds of food we are prone to eat and the illness resulting from it, we can conclude that if we eat foods that are more nutritious, we should be able to experience better health outcomes because of it.

So what exactly can we consider real food? Basically, anything that walks, flies, swims, or is grown is what God created for consumption to sustain our bodies. If we stay within this realm in terms of what we eat, the battle is partially won. What we're left with is the preparation of food and what gets added to it that creates a negative impact.

Modern nutritional science is relatively young, dating back to less than a hundred years ago, when vitamins were first isolated and synthesized for use in the treatment of certain nutritional deficiency-related diseases. Scientists are constantly gaining new information about the human body and its metabolic functions, thanks to new technology and more in-depth studies. And as a result, nutrition scientists are constantly updating the available "facts" based on findings from the latest clinical trials.

However, because the system is not geared toward prevention, the latest information from the nutritional health community doesn't make its way to implementation into the health-care mindset. Rather, it seems locked into the mode of identifying the disease that is triggering a particular symptom, then prescribing a drug to mitigate it—disease care. Medical schools train doctors to treat patients in this way, and the vast majority receive no instruction in nutrition. In fact, doctors are only now being taught about nutrition as a benefit to patient health and wellness.

I remember attending my first conference as a certified health coach. I had been certified by a very reputable nutrition school, so I naively assumed that everyone thought like I did. There were very few breakout sessions that had anything to do with prevention or nutrition, so I made it a point to attend each one on the schedule that did. I attended a session relevant to nutrition where one of the doctors on the panel had gotten his undergraduate degree at Tulane University in New Orleans. When he revealed that his B.S. degree was in Culinary Medicine, I was so inspired to learn that such a program even existed it was like music to my ears.

Even though it was one of a few such pre-med curriculums of its kind in the entire nation, at least it was a sign of hope. It was reassuring to know that Tulane University's medical school understood the importance of training their future doctors to assist their patients with diet and lifestyle modifications.

Too often people develop a mindset that relies on medication to address only the symptoms, when focusing on prevention would be a much better option. If people train themselves to know the obvious truth that diet and nutrition are the keys to sustained health, we will have fewer problems with obesity and chronic illness beginning with doctors. We'll also have a lot fewer nightstands filled with bottles of pills for people that get sicker, not better.

Most doctors know that they don't really cure diseases their patients have, they mostly treat symptoms. You hear a lot about the frustration doctors feel because their patients don't seem to improve from year to year. Much of it stems from noncompliance on the patient's part, but I believe there is a deeper issue.

Patients don't have a vested interest in their own health outcomes if all they have to do is hit numbers on a lab report. I once had a client tell me that on a rare instance he did go to the doctor because his wife insisted on it. And when his doctor asked his reason for coming in, he told him he just wanted to make sure he wasn't dying!

In the majority of cases, they are simply treating symptoms of an ailment that will eventually run its course. When it comes to colds and flu, the body's immune system defends itself against viruses, including Covid-19. Proper rest, diet, and a strong immune system will enable the body to fight illness and disease. Yet Western medicine with its disease care model, virtually ignores measures that would boost the body's immune system, thus allowing the body to do the fighting for us.

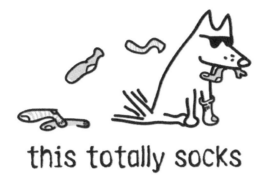

this totally socks

What did the 2020 Pandemic teach us?

We just emerged from a global pandemic where most of the country was shut down for the better part of a year. We were isolated, frustrated, and paranoid for the most part, and we seemed to learn very little about how to fight it or protect ourselves from diseases like it. Bear in mind that the common cold is just another type of coronavirus. Our public health leaders, both local and national, failed to give us any clear path to understanding what we were dealing with, and any useful information that might have come from our health-care sector got swallowed up in a political scrum. A very unfortunate part of the pandemic for Americans was that it happened during an election cycle during which we would be voting for president, which politicized our perception of the coronavirus to the point where we became apathetic to where it even originated. Because of that fact, it has been difficult for the public to discern any real lessons learned.

As it relates to our general health, the pandemic exposed the fact that we are also in the midst of an ongoing international vitamin D deficiency pandemic. A full 70 percent of the world's population is deficient in vitamin D, which is the master key to the human body's immune system. Deficiency in this important nutrient makes us more susceptible to a variety of chronic diseases, such as cancers, viruses, and more. According to the Centers for Disease Control and Prevention (CDC), 70 to 80 percent of all Americans are vitamin D deficient, and blacks and Hispanics are even more deficient because darker skin tone doesn't synthesize UV rays from the sun as well as lighter skin does.

Those that were most vulnerable to the ravages of Covid were in nursing homes, where age, vitamin D deficiency, and obesity put seniors at the greatest risk. When you consider that the average age of death from Covid was 78.6 years, along with vitamin D deficiencies at 82 to 88 percent among this population, it's no surprise their morbidity was highest.

A person who does not work outside is unlikely to receive enough exposure from the sun to get the sufficient amount of vitamin D. When I researched cities in the US with the highest percentage of vitamin D deficiency, I was surprised to learn that they are all the sunshine states like Arizona, California, and New Mexico. The primary reason for this is that people wear protective clothing and sunscreen when out in the sun, which block UVB rays, or they avoid the sun altogether and go outside after the sun goes down.

What the medical profession call cold and flu season is actually low vitamin D season that occurs when the sun doesn't provide sufficient UVB rays. The sun doesn't provide enough UVB during the fall and winter months for people in the world who live above the 35th parallel, so it is necessary to supplement with vitamin D during these months. We learned in high school that cold weather doesn't make us sick, that it's actually viruses that do. Yet we incorrectly believe that the change in the weather condition is the cause. More accurately, it is the change in seasons that diminishes our body's ability to synthesize UVB rays, coupled with a lack of vitamin D supplementation that causes a rise in cold and flu.

With sufficient vitamin D levels, it is safe to assume that most chronic diseases people experience in America would be avoidable, provided they also maintain a lifestyle and diet regimen that supports healthy living. I've seen far too many cases of individuals who suffered from chronic diseases and were taking several medications to treat each one. For some, all it takes is an unexpected brush with death, and suddenly they are willing to make the necessary changes because they want to live. Once you regain your health following an illness, it can be a strong motivator for some men to continue taking an active role in their health journey.

I can attest to that fact from my own personal experience with bladder cancer, yet still others continue to take their health for granted. A daily attitude of gratitude can help you cultivate a positive outlook on life which will help you sustain your life. Unfortunately, for a great many men who have a history of bad habits, finding the discipline required to stay on course is too difficult for them. So they spend the rest of their lives in declining health, leading to a premature death.

When we examine our approach to health behavior, we need to first accept the fact that most of us do not behave in a rational way. It is rational to think that if I give you the right information about how to maintain optimal health, you will simply process the information and act accordingly.

But that's just not how humans behave, and especially men, who like to think they are in control at all times. In reality, they do have the control. But that doesn't result in doing the right thing. With control comes the responsibility to determine our health outcome. What I'm giving you is knowledge that took me years to obtain, but I don't expect you to blindly trust what I say and Just Do It.

The familiar Nike slogan is simplistic, and it certainly doesn't cast a magic spell enabling one to just do it. No, I expect in most cases the slogan to go in one ear, then out the other. As I've told you repeatedly, remember, people (especially men) usually have to reach a pain point before taking action, and even then it's no guarantee. There's a big difference between knowing something better needs to be done, and doing the better thing. The motivation to make positive changes in your life usually has to come from deep within, where you live by the mantra to "contend for your why." Most of us need an unequivocal reason for doing anything significant, like recognizing that not doing it will literally cost you your life. Crossing a railroad track on foot as you see a train headed towards you provides a clear answer for "what is your why?"

Most doctors enter the medical field with a passion for helping people get better, and many despair over the difficulty in creating optimum health outcomes for more of their patients. They give the best advice they know how to give, provide the best medication they can, yet people continue to get sicker. And they feel like they're not really making a difference. The only way we as a nation are going to see substantial improvements in health and health care is by making substantial improvements in our behavior towards health and health care. And that unequivocally involves the patient in a more substantial way.

In Chapter 4, I spoke about Dr. Myles Spar, an integrative medicine physician and the author of *Optimal Men's Health*. I highly recommend that you read it. In this landmark book, he states his bottom line as this: "Achieving optimal health is the most important factor in reaching your goals, and you have many ways to do this besides medications. The approach in this book is an integrative one, based on precision prevention: what can get in the way of staying healthy, and what you can do about it, from diet and exercise to supplements and meditation."

From this quote you can gather that the goal of optimal health is something to strive for, and that it takes some effort and determination, which points to your behavior. Optimal health can be defined as a state of health that focuses on mental health, and healthful relationships, in addition to good nutrition and exercise. So clearly there is a major behavioral component to optimal health. Behavioral economists understand that we are irrational by nature. But recognition of this fact doesn't bring about change.

I've learned to recognize that people are irrational, but in very predictable ways. Understanding this has often given me a slight advantage when I'm coaching someone, so that I stay a couple of steps ahead of them in the health game. An example is when you, my client, turn what should be a health decision into an emotional one.

Let's say you come across a box of Krispy Kreme donuts that someone so thoughtfully left in the breakroom at work, and they had the nerve to set them down right next to a bowl of fresh fruit. You know it would be the right thing to have a piece of fruit instead, but you grab a glazed donut because it's still warm. It's easy to rationalize that you'll eat better tomorrow, but today you deserve to have a donut. Now, I love warm Krispy Kreme glazed donuts as much as the next guy, but they don't love me.

In fact, those Krispy Kreme donuts don't give a damn about me, whether they're warm or not! I could convince myself that having just one would be like getting a warm hug. But I've fallen for that trick enough times to know that the stomachache I'd get from that gooey ring of dough and sugar isn't worth it. Especially considering the fact that I'd invariably eat two, and a few days later I'd be carrying around an extra pound. Living a life of optimal health requires that you constantly make the best choices based on your "why."

> *He who has a why to live for can bear almost any how.* —Nietzsche

U.S. President's Heart Attack Triggers Obesity Epidemic

On September 24, 1955, at age sixty-four, President Dwight D. Eisenhower suffered a massive heart attack while on vacation in Colorado. From that moment on, the nation became obsessed with the issue of heart disease, as the seemingly invincible commander-in-chief ran the free world from his hospital bed at Fitzsimons Army Hospital in Aurora, Colorado. The rugged image of President Eisenhower as a World War II hero couldn't protect him from the cause and effect of a lifestyle and diet that could not sustain his health.

In March 1949, years before suffering a heart attack at age fifty-nine, his friend and personal physician, Major General Howard Snyder advised him that he needed to cut back his four-pack-a-day smoking habit. Eisenhower had begun smoking at West Point as a cadet. After only a few days of limiting his smoking, he decided that counting his cigarettes was worse than not smoking at all, so he quit cold turkey, never having another cigarette the rest of his life. But I surmise the damage had already been done.

At the time of Eisenhower's illness, there was increasing interest in understanding the cause of cardiovascular disease, and although smoking was prevalent in the 1950s, some researchers were looking at dietary causation. After Eisenhower had been hospitalized for a few days on absolute bed rest, doctors decided to consult with noted Harvard cardiologist Paul Dudley White regarding his treatment. Dr. White was one of the leading cardiologists of his time and instructed Eisenhower's attending physicians to get him up out of bed.

As soon as possible, Dr. White had the ailing President sitting up more and doing light exercise, a practice used today because doctors understand that inactivity increases the likelihood of blood clots in arteries leading to the brain. Dr. White also prescribed a diet for Eisenhower that was low in saturated fat and dietary cholesterol and required that the president continue a level of physical activity to control his weight. Eisenhower being very disciplined did exactly as he was told, following the restrictive diet Dr. White prescribed. But his weight increased, and so did his cholesterol. Nonetheless, President Eisenhower recovered from his 1955 massive heart attack and was given a green light to run for reelection by most of his inner circle, except Dr. White.

Ancel Keys, a physiologist from the University of Minnesota and friend of Dr. White's, believed he had the solution. It was cholesterol and saturated fat. Based on his now famous Seven Countries Study, Keys believed that the percent of saturated fat contained in the diets of the seven countries he researched had a direct correlation to their level of coronary heart disease. To this day the findings of his Seven Countries Study are in dispute, where his critics argued that he started out with a study of twenty-two countries, but then cherry-picked the seven that supported his theory.

Although Keys' work continues to shape our beliefs about fat and cholesterol, further analysis of the Seven Countries Study remains significant in the area of animal protein, which has an even stronger association to heart disease today than saturated fat.

The most troubling outcome is that food manufacturers were waiting in the wings with hundreds of processed products that were either fat free or low fat. Their aim? To take advantage of the new information about products that would be perceived as "healthy," hoping to strike it rich with the onset of this paradigm shift in nutrition that changed the landscape in terms of processed foods that would fill our shelves. Sadly, cardiovascular disease, obesity, diabetes, and other diseases have only gotten worse since the government started telling us what to eat.

The new Public Enemy #1 is not fat, but sugar. And the biggest takeaway is that food manufacturers are more interested in selling us foods that we can't seem to get enough of. They know exactly how to keep us coming back for more. The fat was removed from hundreds of foods, making them taste terrible, so they replaced the fat with sugar. You see, we are fighting a battle we have no chance of winning unless we understand we are on our own and need to arm ourselves with the right information.

The pharmaceutical companies are in on the game too. They know that our health-care system is really a disease-care model. So their drugs feed into the notion that doctors are trained to treat symptoms and that we will focus on suppressing each symptom with another drug without concern for prevention or a cure. The goal is to have loyal customers who never get better, dutifully following our doctor's orders to take individual medications for each symptom until we die. It's a great plan if your goal is to make money. But if you want to break the endless cycle, you have to play by a different set of rules. Your own:

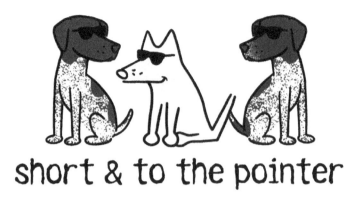

short & to the pointer

Here are some new health rules:

- **Start by getting to know yourself better**—Your health involves the whole self: body, mind, and spirit. We're all going to die one day, but living the best life you can every day is what winners do. Commit to eating better, moving more, and becoming friends with the man inside your head. You know when you don't feel well physically, so stop doing things to yourself that don't make you feel well and start doing things that do. That voice in your head is yours. Don't ignore what your conscience tells you, especially when you know it's for your own good. Health begins with a positive mindset, and you're the only one in control of that. Be a leader, not a follower, and resolve to finish well.

- **Pull your head up!** Literally. I catch myself doing this too; looking down at my cell phone when what I need to do is hold my hands up high enough so that my neck and spine are in proper alignment. We are part of an entire generation who will be suffering from chronic neck and back pain as we age, and it will be because of these so-called smartphones. And most of the time, what are we looking at on our smartphones? Most likely it's just junk food for the eyes or even worse, our minds! The term "smartphone" couldn't be more ironic because the phone might be smart, but it's certainly not making us any smarter. Look up at the sky every now and then, and appreciate it when you see it. Look up at the person in the grocery store checkout and give that person a smile. Even if you're wearing a mask. Chances are, it will show in your eyes, and you'll get a smile back. Give it a try! Making eye contact is a form of nourishment that the age of smartphones and Covid isolation has robbed us of. We will eventually get back to some sense of human normalcy, and we'll have to relearn a few things. Start practicing them now.

- **Get to know your chiropractor**—Most people are either ignorant or skeptical of chiropractors. Those that do use them, do so only if they have a major problem with their neck or back due to a car accident or something similar. But chiropractic care has a long history of bringing relief to even mild chronic pain, and even saving lives, despite opposing views from practitioners of Western medicine. Chiropractic visits should be part of your healthy lifestyle and here's why. The list of benefits from chiropractic care is indeed long, ranging from relief from back pain, neck pain, muscle tension, and headaches, to increasing energy, lowering blood pressure, improving digestion, and promoting healing and recovery, just to name a few. And this is by no means an exhaustive list! My colleague Dr. Tyra Beavers gave an extensive interview about the benefits of chiropractic care, and you can read the transcript in the last section, "In Their Own Words."

In terms of modern chiropractic, Daniel David Palmer is widely credited with having given the first chiropractic adjustments in 1895. An interesting point to know is that doctors in Persia and other parts of the ancient world were performing spinal manipulations as far back as 1000 A.D. A graphic illustration depicting this type of procedure is contained in one of the five volumes of Avicenna's *Canon of Medicine*, the most authoritative medical text in the Islamic world at the time. In *The Official History of Chiropractic in Texas,* by Walter R. Rhodes, statistical records reveal the number of influenza cases documented nationwide during the Spanish flu outbreak of 1917–1918, and how chiropractors played an important role in saving thousands of lives during the world's deadliest pandemic. National figures showed that 1,142 chiropractors treated 46,394 patients for influenza during 1918, with a loss of only 54 patients—one out of every 886. These patients had been given up for dead by traditional medical doctors, but chiropractors stepped in and started giving treatments to these at-risk patients, and the vast majority of them survived.

- **Eat mostly whole foods**—This means foods close to their natural state, such as fresh vegetables, fruits (not fruit juice!), leafy greens, and whole grains. Lean meats are best, and eat fatty meats in moderation. Foods that come in a box, bag, or can are considered processed foods, meaning the structure was altered to some degree to extend their shelf life, and oftentimes sugar was added. Bisphenol or BPA is a plastic coating that lines the inside of most cans. Unless it's marked low sodium, the preservative salt is used. Also, low-quality food is used in cans. Eat these foods in moderation. Most frozen vegetables are acceptable because they are minimally processed. Healthy whole grains, such as brown rice, wheat berries, barley, farro, steel cut oats, are great alternatives to refined carbs like pastas and white rice. Treat fat-free foods like they were poison. Fat-free foods have loads of added sugar to compensate for the loss of taste. Some fat is good for the body if it's the right kind.

- **Sugar is poison**—Glucose is our body's energy source, but too much sugar can literally kill you. It raises your risk for Type 2 diabetes, heart disease, cancer, obesity, and even Alzheimer's. Don't drink sugary beverages like soda, sweetened tea, sports drinks, and especially all those fancy coffee drinks. Do all you can to drastically reduce the sugar in your diet. There are a lot of artificial sweeteners on the market, and they all profess to help you lose weight. We may reduce calories and even lose some weight with artificial sweeteners, but they trick you into thinking you can have all you want. In addition to the psychological disadvantages, a new study finds that artificial sweeteners can damage the healthy bacteria in your gut. There are a few natural sweeteners on the market that don't add calories. Two that I would recommend are monk fruit, and stevia. Eating natural foods that have sugar, like carrots, berries, beets, sweet potatoes and more, will crowd out the sugar cravings and give your body the energy it needs.

- Not all fat is bad for you—As a matter of fact, when the entire food industry went fat-free, we got fatter! Why? Because when the American Heart Association, and the Food & Drug Administration told us all saturated fats were bad for us, food manufacturers, jumping on the bandwagon, removed the fat from our food. But processed foods taste awful without the fat. So they added sugar to compensate, and our diets have been negatively affected ever since. Healthy fat gives you satiety, a sense of feeling full-such as in eating avocado, raw nuts, fatty fish like mackerel, sardines, wild salmon, olive oil, grass-fed red meat, coconut oils, and even butter from grass-fed cows. Lean fatty proteins like organic chicken, pork (advertised by meat packers as the "new white meat"), and organic chicken are excellent diet staples, but always practice moderation.

As you age, you should literally treat animal proteins more like a garnish, and have a predominance of plant-based foods on your plate. Lots of leafy greens and vegetables resembling the colors of the rainbow will serve you well.

- **Stay hydrated**—Drink clean, fresh water mostly. And if you drink alcohol, no more than two per day and don't drink every day. At a minimum let there be at least two days in a row where you do not drink any alcohol, and on those days drink an abundance of water to flush your system of toxins.

- **Boost your immune system**—When the Covid-19 pandemic struck, everyone rushed out to buy toilet paper. We all need toilet paper, but we should have rushed out to buy a supply of Vitamin D3 first, because this is one of the best ways to support the body's immune system. Dr. Stephen Fauci let it slip that he himself took 8,000 to 9,000 IUs a day of vitamin D for that reason, but he seemed to stress more the importance of wearing masks even after being vaccinated, rather than telling us to keep our vitamin D levels optimal. Approximately 80 percent of Americans are immune suppressed, needing vitamin D supplementation. There's a very useful app called *"dminder"* that will teach you how to get optimal levels of vitamin D from the sun's UVB rays, and tell you whether you need to supplement during the fall and winter months when UVB rays from the sun are not available.

- **Stress kills**—Constant stress prevents you from losing weight. Stress causes your body to be flooded with an alarm system hormone called cortisol. Cortisol is a fat blocker, meaning it prevents you from releasing fat because the body might need it as an emergency source of energy. Fat is one of the body's sources of energy, but storing too much of it can be harmful to your body. The main takeaway here is that stress can wreck your immune system more than anything; therefore, you must learn to regulate it. Learn how to meditate. Sitting in a lotus position might look a little silly, it might even feel silly. But I'm certain you'd rather do that than be lying in a hospital bed. I'm dead serious!

- **Practice Healthy Masculinity**—Start embracing your masculinity in a way that is healthy and productive. The traits that push men to take foolish risks or engage in bad behavior, also drive men to be heroic. You can be a hero to your little daughter by accepting her invitation to a tea party on the floor in the playroom. Your little girl will still look to you for protection from thunder and lightning! It takes a real man to go shopping with his wife, and even hold her purse while she rifles through a clothes rack. On the rare occasion that my wife can get me to go shopping with her, I sometimes come across another manly man in a department store holding his wife's purse, and I'll whisper, "Nice bag, fella!" as we pass. Obviously, neither one of us feels less than a man; in fact, we exemplify a quiet, manly confidence that is unshakeable. Masculinity is never threatened; it is quiet, and confident. And the one person that knows you're a real man is your woman! Break all the rules by setting new ones.

CHAPTER 6

Treat Your Body Like You Do Your Car

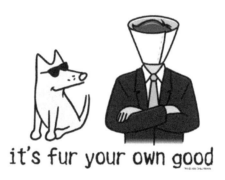

it's fur your own good

Generalizations abound about the way most men take their health for granted, to the point that men themselves accept the perception as a foregone conclusion, even though we're not all guilty. I've chosen another generalization—men's affinity for automobiles—to illustrate several points about male behavior that can have a negative impact on their health. Through analogy, we can take cues from men's relationship to their automobiles and apply it their body—in the hope of adopting better behaviors that result in improved health outcomes.

You'll recall, in Chapter 4, the quote from Dr. Ash Tewari, who was serious in saying he believed that men take better care of their cars than their bodies. Dr. Tewari sees firsthand the toll personal health neglect takes, and he is passionate in his quest to save the lives of men who would otherwise wait too long to finally address issues that could have been treated much earlier, with more-positive outcomes. As with thousands of other practitioners in his field, Dr. Tewari's message to all US men is to be proactive about their health, and literally treat their bodies at least as well as they treat their car. And to that goal, I might add that each man should reach out to other men with the same message. So in the nomenclature of automobiles and how they should be cared for in order to stay on the road, let's examine some analogies that might bring awareness to what's threatening our endangered male species.

Use your Automobile Club Card

Whenever your car breaks down in the middle of nowhere, what's the first thing you do? If you're like me, you reach into your wallet and pull out the second most valuable card in it, your Automobile Club of Southern California membership card, or Triple A as it's commonly known! I wouldn't be surprised if you already have the phone number stored in your smartphone. By the way, in case you're wondering, the most valuable card in your wallet is your driver license! And when you apply this analogy to your health, imagine having a pain in your foot and you limp around for weeks, hoping it will go away. You don't know exactly what it is and you're a little afraid to ask. The question is, how long are you willing to wait this out, especially when the pain is progressively worse, and your anxiety is increasing?

That's when it's time to use your Triple A mindset and call a doctor. In this case, a podiatrist, but if you have only a primary care doctor, then that doctor will gladly refer you to one. However, a CDC survey among men revealed that 23 percent of white men say they don't have a regular doctor, while 31 percent of blacks, 47 percent of Hispanics, 30 percent of Asians, and 36 percent of Native Americans and Alaskan natives also don't have a regular doctor.

These days, it's easier to save yourself a trip by having a video-conference online with your doctor, thanks to our new Covid protocols, or just jump on a phone call.

This task is not a hard one, but too often men will make it seem like it is. If you find yourself doing that, I want you to realize and admit that you're just being lazy, and it's only going to cause you more needless suffering as your condition worsens. There could be any number of things wrong with your foot, but you won't know until you go. I've heard of situations where a guy's had a broken toe or an infection, a case of gout, or in my case plantar fasciitis. These are all very treatable conditions that could get much worse if you ignore them, so don't!

Plantar fasciitis is basically inflammation of the fibrous tissue that runs along the bottom of the foot, which connects the heel bone to your toes. It hurts like hell, trust me. But it can be treated. Gout, which is fairly common, is a form of inflammatory arthritis that can be triggered by certain foods, like red meat, scallops, turkey, liver, and especially beer! A little knowledge can go a long way, but then when you get the knowledge, get some help. You don't need to suffer in silence!

Chiropractic Works!

If you'll recall, before I became a full-time health coach, I helped open a brand-new restaurant for Elon Musk at his SpaceX rocket factory in Hawthorne, California. Working long hours for months, I came down with a pretty serious case of plantar fasciitis just prior to my departing SpaceX to begin my health coaching career. I limped around for two weeks as the pain progressed, before I decided to take some time off and make an appointment with a podiatrist, who promptly diagnosed my condition. I'd never heard of plantar fasciitis, but I was intimately familiar with its symptoms by now. The pain centered near the heel of my left foot, and it was excruciating. I was literally crippled. The pain was always more pronounced first thing in the morning. I had a whole ritual of sitting up on the side of the bed first with both feet on the floor; then I would stand up my good foot and gingerly touch the other foot to the floor. Once the pain subsided from the blood flow, I would hobble off to begin my day of limping.

The podiatrist told me that I would likely need surgery if the treatments he was recommending didn't improve my situation. After taking a mold of my feet, he ordered a pair of custom-made orthotics that I was to wear every day. He prescribed a couple of physical therapies and stretches that might help, in addition to an anti-inflammatory medication I had to take for a couple of weeks. One of the therapies he recommended was to take a small frozen water bottle and roll my stockinged foot over it a couple of times a day, along with some leg stretching exercises. After a week or so I saw very little progress, so I became resigned to the fact I would need surgery.

As a last-ditch effort I decided to get a second opinion, so I went to see a chiropractor my wife recommended. Now, I'd been to a chiropractor before for a neck and shoulder issue years ago, but I had no idea how she would be able to help me with this particular problem. I was desperate, so I agreed to go because I was willing to try anything. Little did I know that the source of my problem turned out to be my hip, which was noticeably misaligned, and it took my chiropractor, Dr. Tyra Beavers, about three minutes to diagnose the real issue.

Dr. Beavers had me lie back on the treatment table and put my feet together, at which point she could see right away that one of my legs was shorter than the other. Even I could see it! A couple of quick adjustments to align my hip, and both my feet were magically the same length again. Dr. Beavers also noticed that my feet were slightly overpronated, which means they both roll inward when I walk, making me mildly flat-footed. The orthotics I was wearing at the time were helping correct my slightly flat feet. After some very interesting adjustments to the numerous bones in my feet, I stood up and felt like a new man!

That's when I heard for the first time the delightful little song, "Chiropractic works!" sung by Dr. Beavers to the tune of "Nah, nah, nah, nah, nah"! It took a couple more visits getting the same adjustment to keep me in alignment, because my body had gotten used to being in that misaligned state for so long. But I was well on the way to recovery as my body gradually got used to being properly aligned again. Because my chef chores required me to be on my feet most of the day, it took several weeks for the inflammation to go down.

But at least I was able to continue working on my feet. To this day, because my orthotics give my arches support, I wear them whenever I wear shoes, but I'm happy to report that my plantar fasciitis is completely healed. If I hadn't reached out for help when my heel was first afflicted, the outcome would have been much worse. Can you say, needless surgery?

About a year after meeting with Dr. Beavers, I left SpaceX and joined her practice as her very first health coach. It was a perfect fit, and in the transition I learned that thousands of health coaches across the country are an integral part of chiropractic practices. Unlike in a medical doctor's office or a clinic, many chiropractors are trained in specialized areas such as chiropractic physiology, chiropractic nutrition, and diabetes self-management education. As a paraprofessional diabetes educator, it turned out to be an ideal environment to work in because there is a high percentage of people we see

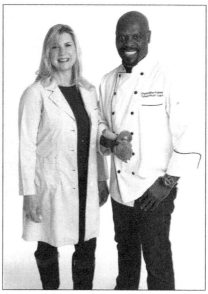

Tyra Beavers, DC and Health Coach LaRue Palmer (2017)

who are either prediabetic or diabetic. People also benefit from my extensive nutrition knowledge that helps anyone looking to lose weight naturally and safely. Many areas of health coaching are becoming highly specialized, which is why board certification will soon be available for those that want to take their credentials to a higher level.

Here's a free chiropractic tip: According to Dr. Beavers, the Covid lockdown resulted in a lot of people suffering from foot issues because so many were not wearing shoes day in and day out— opting to walk around barefoot. It's not good to walk around barefooted all the time, and most people could benefit from wearing arch-supporting insoles.

Don't ignore the check engine light

This brings me to another car analogy: that annoying amber light that appears on your dashboard to alert you that some type of maintenance is required. And you know that light won't go away until you take your car to a mechanic. That *check engine* light is an early warning sign that some issue with your vehicle needs to be addressed. It could be as serious as an oil leak in your timing cover that can cost you about $2,500 to repair, or something much less serious like an oil change, which can run you about $50 in most cars. We don't have the luxury of a check engine light for our bodies, but we do get warning signs in the form of symptoms. And we should all have sense enough to know we should make periodic visits to the doctor, who will give us a multipoint service inspection like mechanics do for a used car.

One reason there is a gender health gap (elaborated on in Chapter 2) is the different behavior response between men and women when symptoms do arise. In most cases, women will notice even a slight change in their bodies that serves as an early warning, but most men will instinctively come up with any number of reasons to simply let it go, until they can't ignore it any longer. Those same men will dutifully take their car in when that *check engine* light comes on. Men will, thinking of saving money and trouble later, get a timely repair on their car. That scenario of ignoring your body's check engine light is so typical and so predictable, but so unnecessary. Yet men are known for it. Can someone please tell me why?

Guys, it goes without saying but I'm going to say it anyway: when you feel something unusual in your body and it persists for longer than what would be considered a reasonable period of time, just as a precaution make an appointment with your doctor and have him or her check you out. If it is a rare case of indigestion that goes away, you can skip the doctor appointment. You might have to wait to get an appointment anyway, and your symptoms could improve. But if it's something that occurs so frequently that you have to keep a supply of Mylanta on hand at all times, then definitely have it checked out. Digestive issues that are masked with over-the-counter (OTC) remedies are a sign of major trouble ahead.

I have a cherished client named Raina, who is a longtime patient of Dr. Beavers. I became her health coach shortly after joining Dr. Beavers' practice. This gave me the unique opportunity to help her start a healthy diet regimen, and at the same time monitor her health progression as she aged gracefully. Raina was seventy-nine at the time I started coaching her, and she would come to the office for in-person treatment. When she first started treatment with Dr. Beavers, she was suffering from joint stiffness, poor posture, and loss of hearing. To see her today, you would have to say she is a true medical miracle.

At the beginning of our coaching relationship, she would exclaim about how beneficial her sessions were, and that her husband Alan could also benefit from working with me. Months went by and Raina was getting good nutrition coaching, while continuing to receive regular massages, stretching and flexibility treatments, plus spinal adjustments as needed. In time, Raina began to show remarkable improvement. Miraculously, the treatment improved her posture noticeably, as she was a rather tall woman. Her balance, range of motion and flexibility increased, and the spinal adjustments even improved her hearing. Other patients used to often complain about how loud she spoke during her treatments because she couldn't hear herself. Over time she was able to modulate to a softer speaking voice because she was able to hear better, all benefits from consistent chiropractic care.

It wasn't long before Alan ended up in the hospital with very serious digestive issues. Raina spoke out to him often about how he needed to improve his diet, or he would end up sick. Alan's favorite food was pizza, and he didn't care much for vegetables. When I finally met him for the first time, it was at his bedside at home after he was released from hospital. From that point on, I've continued to make biweekly house visits, taking care of their grocery shopping and preparing home-cooked meals, while monitoring their health progress. Dr. Beavers makes house calls as well to keep Raina in good shape.

One day I was driving near their home in the Hollywood Hills, so I decided to pay them an unscheduled visit. I needed to do an inventory of their pantry and kitchen prior to my cooking day. When I arrived at their home, I saw a bottle of Mylanta on the kitchen counter, which gave me no cause for alarm. But later when I saw an entire case of Mylanta in the garage, I had to speak up. I nonchalantly grabbed the bottle on the counter and asked Alan, "Who's been using this?" And without a care in the world, Alan said, "Oh, that would be me. My doctor said it was fine to use as needed for occasional heartburn." When I asked him

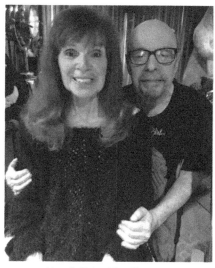

Alan & Raina Handleman –
A Chiro-Integrative Health success story

how long he had been using it, he thought for a second and said with a straight face, "Twenty years or so."

At this point I no longer had a straight face. My mouth was wide open.

I said, "Alan, I'm sure the doctor didn't mean for you to just drink this stuff!" As it turns out, nearly every day he was using it, especially when he had pizza, his food of choice. With this revealing piece of information, I had no alternative but to assume that my client definitely had some gut issues, but in order to verify the diagnosis, I ordered a blood test to find out what the cause of his chronic heartburn was, and to what extent. My suspicions were confirmed when his test came back positive for intestinal permeability, which leads to leaky gut syndrome. Alan was probably at the beginning stages of leaky gut syndrome. As of this writing, Alan has yet to respond to my urgings to change his diet and get serious about treating his digestive issues. One day his situation will take a turn, and he'll be forced to deal with a worse situation than he has now. I go through this with a number of my male clients, but that's just how some men are. They only learn things the hard way. Alan's a great guy, so I'm going to keep nagging him until he takes me seriously or gets sick again. It will probably be the latter to be honest, but I'll be there for him even though it will be harder. But it doesn't have to be!

On the other hand, urinary problems are a common occurrence among men past a certain age, and they are not something that should be allowed to persist for too long before addressing. Remember what I shared with you about how during the Covid pandemic lockdown, I started experiencing some very troubling urinary problems? What I thought was a possible urinary tract infection turned out to be bladder cancer! I spoke about how for several weeks I was waking up numerous times during the night to go to the bathroom. I'm talking five or six times, sometimes more! When I went to pee, there was a heightened sense of urgency, but only a small volume each time. This condition is what's known as an overactive bladder. I was also having the same sensations during the day. I usually drink at least sixty-four ounces of water every day, so frequent trips to the bathroom weren't that unusual, but the pressure and burning irritation were unwelcome features.

In case you didn't know this, it's not normal to have pain, pressure, or burning when you urinate. And it's definitely not normal to have to go to the bathroom five or six times a night. I'm positive that some of the men reading this right now are going through those very symptoms. Some men are embarrassed or subconsciously think they're being wimps if they are concerned and want to have this problem evaluated by a doctor. The reality is that it takes courage to set aside your fears of a potentially bad diagnosis and go through with a medical screening to see what's wrong. Being proactive or responsive to changes in your health is the prudent thing to do, and you should recommend this kind of behavior to every man you know; your son if you have one, your father, uncle, or brother. Chances are, they will be hesitant just like you or so many other men who are, but do it anyway. Encourage them to be responsible towards their health and act accordingly when the *check engine* light comes on. Support one another.

Drive it 'til the wheels fall off

This is a figure of speech we've all heard that's always good for a laugh. But it describes what men do to their body by abusing it to the very end, when it's too late to do anything. In this chapter on car analogies, it serves as a warning to not drive your body like an old jalopy until it nearly or literally won't run anymore. If so, in real life what's likely to happen is that you won't die, but you will become dependent on someone else to take care of you because you didn't have the sense enough to take care of yourself. I know that's harsh, but the truth can be harsh. It's also a harsh reality for whomever would have to become your caretaker. And they would likely be in the position to know that you lived your life without a care in the world about taking care of your health, despite the fact they probably encouraged you to do so, to no avail.

While in college, I drove my 1966 VW Beetle to the point where it had to be towed away. I put a ton of miles on that car in five years, and when I bought it from my girlfriend's brother it had already clocked forty thousand miles. That car was in prime condition when I bought it, but on a student athlete's income, I couldn't afford to keep up on the maintenance. I attended to the bare minimum of items, like gas, brakes, tune ups, oil and tires. But when the more expensive issues arose, I decided to hope and pray they would go away.

Although it's just a figure of speech, without a consistent schedule of maintenance that is adhered to, you can literally drive your car until everything I mentioned breaks down, including the motor! In terms of human health, we call this premature aging. It's easy to understand the concept of premature aging when it comes to an automobile, but for some reason the same logic escapes men when they start feeling the effects of aging but don't do anything to stop it.

Imagine putting a teaspoon of sugar in your gas tank each time you fill it up. Over time, that sugar would have a negative impact on your car. You might be able to drive it for a while without noticing it, but eventually the car's performance would get worse and worse, until it would just stop running altogether. That's exactly what happens to our bodies when we continue to feed it substandard, processed foods and sugary beverages: the predictable outcome is premature aging and an early death. The saddest part is that the human body is engineered to sustain itself, providing we give it the proper fuel, exercise, and rest it needs. Unfortunately, for millions of men that's too much to ask, so they end up suffering needlessly, and if they have a family, their loved ones suffer along with them, in addition to witnessing their heartbreaking decline. In the end they feel cheated, robbed of your most precious gift—time with you. Not a very manly thing to do.

As I write this, I can't help but recall a man I desperately tried to help, who retired at fifty-five, only to spend that retirement sick, depressed, unable to care for himself. He ended up being shuttled between family members as they juggled their own lives, while trying to provide the best situation for him. This man ended up having to live with his elderly mother, who had already done her part to raise him, and now as a full-grown man, when he was disabled by a lifestyle disease of his own doing, she was spending her twilight years caring for him. It became too much for her, so he had to move in with one of his sons. With the son having three young children and a wife, life became difficult for all of them. It was at this point that I tried to intervene. Depression had set in, further complicating the issue and making it impossible for him to see through the fog to motivate himself to get healthy again.

I mentioned earlier that diabetes is a lifestyle disease, which is true in the vast majority of cases if you have Type 2 diabetes. Putting your body into a state where it is constantly secreting the hormone insulin in an effort to normalize your blood sugar is a lifestyle choice that eventually affects your health. Eating a poor diet rich in saturated fat, carbohydrates, alcohol, added sugar, high stress, and little to no exercise is a formula for diabetes. The problem for most people is that they don't understand how diabetes is triggered by this lifestyle, to where the wheels start to fall off! Insulin resistance is a condition where the insulin secreted by your pancreas can't do its job of putting glucose into your body's cells, which have become resistant to it. So the glucose builds up in your bloodstream, causing more insulin to be secreted. Too much insulin in your system is called insulin resistance, which leads to Type 2 diabetes. At this point it becomes necessary for you to use drugs or ultimately insulin injections to force the glucose into your cells for energy, and with this condition comes a litany of other co-morbidities (simultaneous chronic health issues) because of the diabetes.

Even if you see a doctor on a regular basis, most doctors will tell you to watch your sugar when they see the pattern of gradually elevated blood glucose numbers. What is typically happening is that your doctor watches your blood sugar continue to rise, without effectively guiding you on how to manage your blood sugar levels through proper diet and exercise. Once your blood sugar reaches a certain level, above 99 mg/dl, you are given Metformin, the common diabetes medication I've mentioned before, which will help your body keep your blood sugar "under control." At that point, unless you make a radical decision to not rely on drugs that act like a Band Aid to regulate your blood sugar, you have begun a slow decline where the Metformin doses increase until they lose their effectiveness altogether. Then you have to graduate to insulin injections. The insulin injections eventually have to increase until . . . I think you get the picture.

The dirty little secret about Type 2 diabetes is that if caught in its early stages, it is often preventable and even reversible, but doctors are only now learning the lifestyle nature of the disease. More importantly, all the comorbidities of diabetes (such as high blood pressure, heart disease, stroke, and even Alzheimer's in some cases) are likewise avoidable. So what's standing in your way? Big Pharma and the institutions that train our doctors, our medical schools.

For each symptom that pops up, there's a drug to take care of it. Diabetes is progressive, which means a cascade of symptoms is added to the initial ones so that before long, you are taking multiple medications for symptoms that will never go away. They just progress until one of the disease symptoms, or comorbidities, kills you. And it all started with elevated blood sugar. Then the wheels fall off.

So what's the solution? The first is to realize that what you're being told by the American Diabetes Association (ADA), the Food and Drug Administration (FDA), and even the American Heart Association (AHA) is wrong. Second, you've got to understand there is a financial incentive for us all to remain sick. The FDA through the Food Pyramid and its replacement, My Plate, gave us information that was not correct. Fats were vilified, and carbohydrates were elevated, which goes directly against what nutritional science is telling us now in its most recent studies.

When fat was stricken from the American diet and deemed to be evil, food manufacturers replaced it with added sugar to compensate for taste. Carbohydrates, especially refined ones that turn to sugar, are problematic for our health as well. Turning this problem around is going to be a monumental task, because it's difficult for doctors to give up the advice they've been peddling for decades and rethink their approach to health. We have a disease-care model, but what we need to develop one day is a health-care model based on prevention of disease.

Take her for a spin

That's what a car dealer will tell you when it's time to test-drive the car you're thinking about buying. But my car analogy implies that you take yourself for a spin. In other words, get outside and move your body in some form of age-appropriate exercise. Yes, it can be boring and seem too much like work, but that's because it is! Going outside is ideal if weather permits, but if not, you can stimulate your body and your mind by getting some movement indoors.

A car left sitting for too long will get a carbon buildup. Moisture will accumulate in areas you don't want that to occur, usually in the oil and crank case. A car needs to be driven every once in a while, so that the engine and its components have a chance to warm up thoroughly, assuring you of optimal performance. This is in addition to regular maintenance. The same holds true for the human body; regular maintenance, and an occasional lap around the track so to speak. In point of fact, to keep your system finely tuned, the body needs much more exercise than your car.

More than that, aging is an obvious risk factor for a number of diseases—like cancer, Alzheimer's, heart disease, stroke, and diabetes. So it's important to keep your body moving, especially if you want to stay independent as you age, while you keep your body properly fueled. As rugged and independent an individual as you think you are right now, if you don't move it you'll lose it! Imagine a time in the not-too-distant future when you'll want to do something as simple as going to the bathroom. What if you have to wait for someone to help you out of your chair, hand you your walker, follow you as you slowly make your way to the bathroom, unbuckle your belt, help you pull down your pants, then ease you down onto the toilet? Provided you can wipe yourself when you're finished, someone will then have to help you get back to your chair! Not a pretty picture, I'll admit.

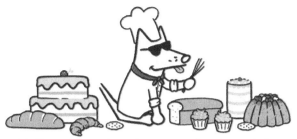

life is what you bake it

There are people right now in their sixties who have to go through this. Because of a debilitating stroke, for example, they can no longer care for themselves. These chronic diseases can be avoided, but they require an attitude of self-preservation, and monitoring situations like hypertension or diabetes that if left unchecked will get worse. Don't think it can't happen to you; it can and does. Treat your body well now and it will serve you later. This isn't hard to figure out, guys. We just suffer from what I've mentioned before, present bias, without regard for the future. Part of it is human nature, and there's another part that I call the superman syndrome, that men seem to be stricken with. It starts when you're young when you've convinced yourself that you're indestructible. But then kryptonite shows up out of nowhere. It's called aging. Medical science has progressed to the point where we can sustain our lives far beyond what humans could a few short decades ago. But it takes in addition incorporating some common sense to live long and prosper, as Mr. Spock says. So I urge you to live wisely in your actions and mindset, and you will die youthful at an old age!

Look for the best mechanic

Once you decide to do something about that *check engine* light in your car, clearly you won't just settle for the first mechanic that comes up on the internet, or a garage you just happened to pass by on your way to the store, will you? Of course not! If you don't have a regular mechanic, you're likely to be online trying to find customer reviews on Yelp, or asking a trusted friend for a referral. The same should hold true when you need a doctor to check you out. Doctors get reviewed too, especially if they belong to a medical group and you have to choose from a long list. Their photograph might be shown; their background and education are listed, along with their areas of specialty. You'll want to make an informed decision with the data you've been provided.

Remember, treat your body as well as you do your car, or hope-fully better. You can buy another car if the one you currently drive can't be fixed, but you only get one body. When you wear that one out, game over. Even when we abuse our body from time to time, they've been engineered to heal themselves, and with a little help can maintain themselves for a long time. Choose the right doctor to be on your health-care team, and when you do, keep him or her accountable. It's a good idea to have a health advocate, someone you trust who will serve as a second-opinion person. That could be your spouse, a trusted relative, or a male friend, someone who cares about you and will speak up on your behalf.

Doctors are often overwhelmed, especially when you consider the shortage of doctors we have. There's never a shortage of patients, because people too often leave their health and well-being up to doctors who already have too many patients. This is why I tell my clients to take responsibility for their own health, so they can stay out of the broken health-care system as long as possible. With all the administrative demands put on doctors—ranging from procedural compliance to accountability and liability issues—the squeaky wheel always gets the grease. So don't be afraid to speak up when you don't feel you're getting all your questions answered to your satisfaction. You be the squeaky wheel, even if you are the only one who sees it that way. And if you have to, fire your doctor and find a better one!

Consult the Owner Manual

In today's information age, the internet is the human equivalent of an owner manual. Any unusual rash, growth, or symptom will send some people to their smartphone or keyboard to consult WebMD to diagnose and perhaps treat what ails them. Doing your own research is a reasonable first step because you can gain some general knowledge about your body and its various parts, but then always consult with your doctor. Never attempt to diagnose something that might be serious. The owner manual for your car can help you locate the gas cap, or find out how to reset the dashboard clock. You wouldn't consult a mechanic to help you with that. There are lots of useful tips and information contained in those owner manuals, just like there are useful basic health tips on the WebMD. But unless you trust the source, the internet can also be a very dangerous place to get information.

For example, if your primary care physician has an affiliate website that can direct you to some curated information they want you to have, then that's the best way to go. These sites are password protected and user friendly, and their purpose is to educate you, the patient. They also allow you the opportunity to communicate with your physician so that you can ask specific questions from the privacy of your computer or smartphone. One of the best features of these health platforms is the ability to have a video conference with your health-care team. Telehealth portals gained prominence during the Covid pandemic, even though some health-care providers were already using them prior to the pandemic. There were a number of silver linings in the pandemic that came to light, and I'm confident that many of them will remain in effect, now that we've moved past the worst of it for the most part.

Moving forward, I'm happy to see that more people have become accustomed to seeking advice through technology. Prior to the pandemic I was seeing 50 percent of my clients in person, about 40 percent through my telehealth portal, and the rest by telephone. I'm confident that in the next couple of years I will be seeing the vast majority of my clients through videoconferencing, which will also enable me to do more group coaching, as people are already getting accustomed to it. Seeing faces and being able to read even limited body language is very helpful in communication, and the technological interaction allows me to use digital diagrams, charts, and videos on-screen.

The Appeal of a Classic Car

If you were to ask a hundred car enthusiasts what defines a classic car, you'd get a thousand different answers. One common answer is that it would have to be at least twenty-five years old. With that as a basic criterion, we would all qualify. And as we reflect on the classic car/human-body analogy I've discussed; we can all agree that what we know about how classic cars are treated—they get pampered by their owners and as a result look as good as they did the day they came off the assembly line.

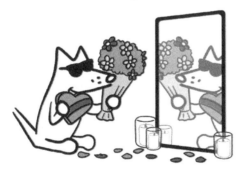

I'm dating myself

None of us is going to look as good as the day we came off the assembly line, because we were babies then. So, let's start from the classic car age determination of twenty-five years old for comparison. When we're twenty-five years old and in the prime of life, we think we're bulletproof. But what are a lot of guys doing between the ages of eighteen and twenty-five? Many of them are engaged in risky behaviors, such as drinking too much, experimenting with drugs, driving too fast, chasing women in excess, playing contact sports, taking high-risk jobs, and playing with guns. Statistics tell us that. You may not have done all of it, but I'm sure most of us were doing some of it. Why do you think our insurance rates start to decline once we pass the age of twenty-five?

Again, statistics show that we start maturing, settling down, and beginning to get our act together a little. Mind you, I said beginning. It usually takes another ten years before the majority of us realize toxic male behavior is unsustainable. By age thirty-five we're well established in a job or career hopefully, many of us blessed to even have started a family. That's when the stakes get much higher, but as I've discussed in this book, we still act as though proper care and maintenance of our bodies is for the health nuts who do yoga and eat kale!

With great advancement in medical science, pharmaceuticals and gerontology (the study of aging), people are living longer. The question, is what will your quality of life be? It starts with a mindset that says you are determined to live well for as long as possible, and then the choices you make will be guided by that determination. As it turns out, we don't suffer from a knowledge deficit. There's plenty of information out there, much of it we know intrinsically. What we suffer from is a behavior deficit, one that prevents us from making sound choices most of the time.

I admire the research that Dr. David Asch is doing in the area of innovative health care and behavioral economics. Dr. Asch is Executive Director of the Penn Medicine Center for Health Care Innovation. He believes that supporting our health with good nutrition is obviously the first line of defense; bearing in mind that we cannot avoid contamination through the environment, so we have to arm our body for that fight. One of his favorite quotes is from a comedian of all things:

> *Hard work pays off in the future, but laziness pays off right now!*
> —Steven Wright

This quote further defines what I alluded to as *present bias*. Perhaps it helps to visualize this line of thinking in another way. Millions of people spend their hard-earned money on state lotteries. Some in the hope of striking it rich for a worthy cause, others just so they can stop working and enjoy the *good life*, while still others are told by lobbyists that it's a great way to support public schools "for the children." I can only speak for my state of California, where our schools continue to suffer from a lack of adequate funding, while the administrators line their pockets. You can play lotteries every day of the week. Just pop into any gas station, grocery, or liquor store.

Humans in general tend to overestimate the likelihood of small probabilities, which is what winning any state lottery is: a small probability. Someone came up with a brilliant slogan and put it on a bumper sticker that said: "State lotteries are a special tax on people who can't do math!" It's not that we can't do the math, we can't feel the math.

When my clients are struggling with cravings and food choices early in their health journey, I tell them that the double cheeseburger with onion rings and a large orange soda won't harm you any more than the grilled chicken and avocado salad will benefit you in the short term. Go ahead and enjoy life and have a cheeseburger *every once in a while*. But most of the time, do what's right for your health. Your body will tell you if you made the right call.

Hopefully, you won't go through life thinking you have to be on a diet every day of your life. You and millions of others have proven that diets don't work. And when you fall off the wagon, don't stay on the ground. And when you find yourself in your man cave, make sure it's a man cave of health!

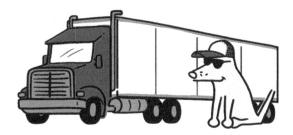

In it for the long haul

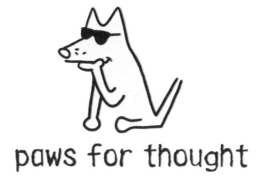

paws for thought

Interviews

In Their Own Words

With Amit Gupta, MD

Following is a transcript of a recent conversation I had with my urologist, Dr. Gupta, MD-MPH. He is an associate professor with Samuel Oschin Cancer Center (part of Cedars-Sinai Medical Center) in Los Angeles. As recounted in Chapter 1 ("A Perfect Example"), I had the good fortune to be treated by Dr. Gupta when my primary care physician, Dr. Daniel Stone, referred me to him. As it turns out, I had Stage 1 bladder cancer, which though low on the cancer spectrum, is an aggressive cancer that has about a 50 percent chance of recurring within the first five years after diagnosis.

As you'll recall, while writing this book during the Covid-pandemic lockdown, I began experiencing symptoms consistent with bladder cancer, which were a frequent need to urinate, a persistent sense of urgency, and at times varying degrees of discoloration in my urine. There was a period when the discoloration cleared up, but when it returned along with the persistent urgency to urinate, I decided Covid or not it was time to get in contact with my primary care physician, Dr. Stone. I was in no position to continue guessing what might be wrong or hoping for my symptoms to clear up. Dr. Stone was not available, so the doctor on call arranged for a video conference.

Initially, by video conference, Dr. Violano instructed me to have my blood and urine tested before attempting to schedule an in-person appointment with a urologist. The results came back positive for some type of cancer, but they were inconclusive as to exactly what type. The next step was to get a CT scan so that we could gain visibility of what specifically might be going on inside my body. The CT scan confirmed at least one small tumor on the interior of my bladder wall, and with a subsequent cystoscopy Dr. Gupta was able to show me the tumor in real time with the help of a tiny camera invading my bladder. It was a sight I will never forget. I felt like I was peering into an underwater garden!

Following a minimally invasive surgical procedure, it turned out that there were actually four tumors on the bladder wall, along with the presence of cancer in my ureter, a small tube that runs down from one of my kidneys and connects to the bladder.

While at a follow-up visit concerning a recent surgical procedure, I asked Dr. Gupta a few questions regarding my particular condition, and how common it was for men he sees in his practice to experience the same thing as I did. I also wanted to know his perspective about the phenomenon of middle-aged men who delay seeking treatment for relatively minor symptoms and the end result of that delay.

LaRue: Dr. Gupta, since I was diagnosed last November with bladder cancer, a number of people including personal friends have indicated that they've experienced some of the same symptoms I presented to you. The odd thing is, they remain hesitant to have their symptoms checked out, even though they are aware of what I went through. One very close friend let his condition get much worse over time, and he ended up being diagnosed with Stage 4 bladder cancer. I imagine you see patients that have delayed getting treatment until they are forced to see a doctor because their symptoms are so much worse. Is it normal for men to wait to seek treatment until it's unbearable?

Dr. Gupta: It's not unusual for men to recognize there is a problem, but they hope it will pass. The bleeding may occur for a while, then stops. The result is that they end up bleeding much more frequently, and that's when they come to see me. And by that time the tumor, which would have been this small last year, is much bigger and needs much more treatment. Or it could have become incurable. So it's a very common thing that men ignore these symptoms. And if they see blood in their urine, they just ignore it and wish it will go away; they think it could be an infection and just ignore it. The delay in diagnosis is very common, and this is an aggressive cancer where the more time they give to it, the more it grows and the more it can spread.

LaRue: I see. So on the front end is the cancer more aggressive?

Dr. Gupta: It's just a more aggressive cancer. Now, there are lots of variations within bladder cancer; there are less-aggressive variants and there are more aggressive variants, but we don't know that up front. I guess the main message is that if a man sees blood in his urine, he should treat it like an urgent situation and see somebody, rather than wait. And even if it goes away, it doesn't mean there is no problem, because a tumor bleeds inter-mittently. It will bleed; then it will stop. It may stop for months before bleeding again. So if you ever see blood, it needs to be looked into.

LaRue: This is no joke!

Dr. Gupta: It's not. And blood in the urine is not just due to bladder cancer. It could be due to kidney cancer. It could be due to kidney stones. It could be a big prostate that can be bleeding. So, not every man that has blood in their urine has bladder cancer; in fact, very few do. But they may have other things, such as a kidney tumor or a big stone in the kidney. All of those need to be diagnosed and fixed before you have a much bigger problem.

LaRue: So what you're telling me is that you can present with one symptom like blood or discoloration in the urine and it could be one of several different conditions, with bladder cancer being the least likely?

Dr. Gupta: Yes! Also, the most dangerous types of cancer are bladder and kidney cancer. Those are the two cancers to worry about if not detected early, and then a bunch of things that are noncancerous but still require diagnosis and treatment.

LaRue: Men come to you at different stages of potential illness, depending on how long it has taken them to finally break down and see a doctor. What is the one most common, or likely, condition men should be concerned with when they see discoloration or blood in their urine like I did?

Dr. Gupta: There are variations. For the male patient who is in his sixties and seventies who has been smoking for ten to twenty years, bladder cancer becomes high on that list. The same person who has not been smoking, then a big prostate causing the bleeding becomes higher on the list. So, it kind of varies, but the management is the same. We start by doing a CT scan, and we look in the bladder. The combination of those two procedures tells us exactly what the issue is; then we treat it and take it from there.

With Marilyn Singleton, MD, JD

Dr. Singleton has a unique background that provides useful insight to my book. Typically, from my perspective, race does not factor into one's background, but when you consider the state of our society when she was growing up and when she was educated, the achievements and perspective of this accomplished black woman are both incredible and inspiring. Dr. Singleton is a prolific writer of op-eds on a wide range of topics (marilynsingletonmdjd.com), a recognized authority on health-care policy, medical ethics, culture and society, and politics. She is my go-to source for anything related to health in general, as well as the sociopolitical arena in regard to public health. We had a wide-ranging discussion about men's health.

> LaRue: The mindset of men in my generation is that they will sacrifice their physical health and well-being, while at the same time avoid going to the doctor because they have to go to work. In other words, they can't take time out to go to the doctor (*I've got a job to do*). What is that about?

> Dr. Singleton: Your question begs another question. Is that an excuse? *I have to go to work; I can't go to the doctor?* No, they really don't want to go to the doctor. And there's always the famous cartoon, as though women didn't have

the same problems, of a doctor pulling on a surgical glove with one digit sticking straight up in the air as if to signify to men, *You have to go to the doctor!* That's what people are thinking, but it's the fear of that image that results in men dying younger than they have to. Prostate cancer pops up in forty year-olds; in fact, the younger you are when you get these types of cancers, it seems like the worse the cancer is. So, the going-to-work part—and that's certainly something I'm sure you explore in your book more deeply than I—is it just an excuse, or is it a fact? Yes, of course they really do have to go to work, and find they often don't have time.

I'm reminded of my uncle Herman, who lived in New Jersey; he's long passed now, but when he started his medical practice, he opened up at 5:30 in the morning so that people could go to the doctor on their way to work. Back in those days before insurance and workplace rules, people did not want their employer to know that they had to go to the doctor. That's actually how he built up his practice. It was open at night and in the morning, and even at lunchtime. In New Jersey he lived close to Red Banks, the namesake river, and because he loved to go fishing he'd close up shop in the late morning and go fishing for a couple of hours, then come back and go to work.

His was one of the original patient-based health models that ended up working out very well for the doctor as well. I always remembered him telling me that the guys he saw didn't want their boss to know that they were going to the doctor, and they didn't want to be docked for any time off of work. There was also an unspoken effort to preserve their image of masculinity by pretending to never have a need to see a doctor.

LaRue: That's fascinating insight, and certainly something I pick up on in many men who make that same excuse. And it's a foolish deception when you consider that they are trying to keep up a façade that they don't get sick. It's my view that the culture needs to open its eyes to the fact that men need to be encouraged to make and keep doctor appointments without fear of being ridiculed or thought less of. Men should feel free to go out and take care of their health issues and not think that it will somehow threaten their masculinity. Along with being complicit in this lie, men feel their bodies are machines that never need maintenance. Having a culture of preventive health care would encourage other men to think like that. It's counterintuitive and very strange!

The economy benefits when men have an employer who is sensitive to the idea of preventive health care, because it reduces wage loss and employee downtime due to illness. At the same time, employers stand to lose on the backend. If a man is disincentivized to pay regular visits to a doctor, he runs the risk of paying higher insurance premiums instead of preventive care, and possible premature death.

DR. SINGLETON: It's interesting to hear you describe what sounds to me like the male dilemma. I remember when I first started in private practice, there was another woman in the department, and she said, "Now, remember, if you need a short schedule on a certain day because you want to see your child's school play, tell them you have an appointment with your stockbroker! Today it's considered cool when men go to their kid's soccer games, but when a woman had to go to her child's function, she was forced to lie and say she was doing the manly business thing. The crossover with the sexes is very interesting, but it's the opposite for men.

Now, if that same man today were to say, "Uh, I have to go to the doctor to get my wellness checkup," he might get looked at cross-eyed! It is funny when you start thinking about all these differences and the way people weave through life. Certainly for the woman who doesn't see her child's play because she doesn't want to look like a "girl" at work, it's psychologically damaging. She feels like she's abandoning her child. And for the man who doesn't go to the doctor, it's certainly physically damaging. And as we all know, health is preventive. Let's face it! [Not] treating something after the fact. Of course, sometimes we can't help it because people just get sick no matter how well they have taken care of themselves.

There was a paper that came out of Johns Hopkins a few years ago, that said at least 70 percent of stuff that's wrong with us we can help prevent or attenuate to a great degree by being mindful of healthy eating and lifestyle. Things that are so simple. As someone once said, "Simple things are simple." But it's not simple if your brain isn't going in that direction. And certainly for some black folks, it's not simple. I was thinking of this the other night, walking back from something in a nice neighborhood, and I said to myself: *This is one reason why black folks have so much trouble with hypertension and diabetes.*

If you live in a neighborhood where you're afraid of getting shot if you go out of your front door after sundown, you're not going to do the after-dinner walk. So, when you hear talk about the social determinants of health, I'm not of the belief that the medical sector has hated blacks for years and that's why there's a problem. There are some real neighborhood problems. I grew up in a bad neighborhood, and it's true you don't want to go out after dark, even though exercise is so important.

It's become more prevalent since Covid that exercise is so good for just about everything, especially when trying to boost your body's immunity. But if you can't do that, then you have to do something else. Not everybody can afford a gym membership, and many people are like me, where they don't enjoy going to the gym. I'd much prefer to just go for a walk, but even that became difficult because of the Covid restrictions.

Sometimes that can become an excuse for not exercising and it might end up affecting your health. If you happen to work somewhere where you can walk at lunchtime, you've got to find a way to build that into a routine and make it just as important as whatever else you decided to do at lunchtime.

LaRue: The title of my book was inspired by a program at Mount Sinai Hospital in New York called Man Cave Health. The urology department converted its waiting room into what we would call a modern-day man cave with all the décor of a sports bar, including sports memorabilia, leather chairs, a coffee bar, and a big-screen television.

Dr. Singleton: Oh, how cool! I had not heard of that, but I'm very impressed.

One thing as a woman doctor that I find interesting as you're discussing this is how men feel about going to the doctor. Throughout my career and certainly when I was a young medical student in residence, I found that I was different things to different people. Some older men, in order to be able to tell me everything I asked them in a medical history, chose to see me as kind of a granddaughter figure. It was never going to be a situation like "I'm the nagging wife" as the way to get someone to tell all. Nonetheless, it can be very hard to get people to tell the truth. But the truth is that everybody hides stuff just a little bit, so you work to find a way to get them to accidently blurt it out. Only twice in my fifty years of seeing patients did somebody say they didn't want a woman, which is interesting because back when I was in medical school we only had ten women out of a hundred thirty–some odd, and now half of all doctors are women. Now guys aren't going to have a choice: you get who you get.

LaRue: I've noticed even in urology, the number of women entering that field seems to be growing more than ever! Is that a correct observation?

Dr. Singleton: Absolutely. Which reminds me of a funny little story. During my residency I was a surgery resident for a couple of years, and when I was in my urology rotation in clinic, there was this one guy who came in and said, "So, where's doctor so-and-so?" And I said, "Oh, he's not in clinic today." But I think it was more a case that he just liked him. It wasn't a case of a man-versus-woman thing, so I did what I had to do, and that was that. I never felt that it was a question of competence. In fact, it became a bit of a joke. One day my colleague was walking by with one of his patients I'd taken care of, and he said, "Well, you're just the best doctor west of the Mississippi!" My colleague and I laughed, and he said the guy was just an old drunk. I told him, "Hey, don't make fun of the best compliment I've had so far in my career!"

But I must say I find your book very interesting because I see you as somebody who's coaching people to health, which is so essential. Each person you encounter is going to need something different from you. Some might see you as a wise person who has come up with the best way to deal with an individual's personal health, yet it's not like you're a doctor who's going to write prescriptions for whatever to treat somebody's pneumonia. But whether they want to look at you as the little brother, the big brother, the dad, they should accept that knowledge. And granted, sometimes men accept things better from another man, and sometimes they'd rather their mother tell them. The challenge is having to figure out the right way to transmit and obtain information from people that hits the nail on the head. So many times people won't tell you what the key thing is, and they dance around it. Men are probably worse at that than women; for some reason, they just don't want to open up.

LaRue: Boy, you said it! Welcome to my world. I researched an article for my book that found that men are more likely to prefer a male doctor if and when they do go, but paradoxically are less likely to open up about their symptoms to a male doctor. Researchers found that the reason was, they don't want to show weakness or dependence to another man. And as you already alluded, another reason why this is the case is that a woman is less likely to judge a man in this instance. On the other hand, researchers also found that men who are more honest to female doctors don't fear any lack of masculine status.

We're going to have to end our interview on that thought, but I want to put an exclamation point on your perspective as a female doctor with incredible insight and empathy towards men's health. I appreciate your sharing them with me, and thank you for joining me in the man cave of health!

Dr. Singleton: It's been a real pleasure!

With Tyra Beavers, DC

Dr. Beavers gave me my first break into the health industry—an opportunity to become a health coach in her thriving practice in Beverly Hills, California. This interview will help you understand why you should have a chiropractor in your Man Cave of Health!

> LaRue: Dr. Beavers, what percentage of men do you have or see in your chiropractic practice?

> Dr. Beavers: Thankfully, men seeking chiropractic care is becoming more prevalent, so I would have to say we're at a ratio of about 60 percent for women versus 40 percent for men. We women are pretty good about taking care of ourselves because we've got to run the ship at home, you know. We do a lot of things there, whereas more men are very driven and focused on providing for the family. And sometimes they don't think about themselves or their health. But as I said, I do think it's becoming more prevalent for men to be more concerned for their health, so that 60/40 ratio in my practice is pretty accurate.

> LaRue: I can understand your desire to be a little diplomatic towards men in this interview, but a lot of the men I see and hear about use the

responsibility of having to provide for the family as an excuse to avoid going to see a doctor on a regular basis, much less seeing a chiropractor!

DR. BEAVERS: Well, I think the mindset of men is starting to change. More people are seeking more natural forms of health care, and they would rather not take a pill for what ails them. They realize that pills are just masking the real problem in many cases and not really correcting the problem. I think more and more people are cluing in on the fact that alternative health measures like chiropractic are the way to go.

LARUE: We've spoken before about how people present to you with symptoms of back pain and neck pain, all the usual reasons someone would seek out a chiropractor in the first place, but you mentioned something in an earlier discussion I thought was interesting in light of the COVID lockdown. Would you share with my readers what you found?

DR. BEAVERS: Of course! I was amazed to see more and more patients during the lockdown coming to see me who were suffering from the same lower-extremity problems: pain in the knee, foot, hip, and lower back primarily. I began to ask certain questions of each of these patients, and I came to realize that most people were not wearing shoes during the pandemic. They would get up in the morning, start their day, and just walk around barefoot all day long. And with that kind of behavior, if your arches are not supported well and one or both of them is rolling inwardly (pronated) or rolling outward (supinated), that means you'd be walking around all day with joints that are twisted or torqued. And that can present a big problem after months of doing that. So, my message to everyone is to not walk around barefoot at home. You must wear a supportive type of shoe—a sandal or house shoe. It's really important.

LaRue: That's really a great point. In fact, I have a personal experience related to it. In the spirit of full disclosure to my readers, before I became a colleague of yours I was actually a patient. As I have briefly sketched out earlier in the book, back when I was still working as a chef for Elon Musk at SpaceX, I was diagnosed with plantar fasciitis, which I have since learned is quite common among people who stand for long periods of time and work on hard surfaces. Let me remind the reader that plantar fasciitis symptoms can include a dull or stabbing pain on the bottom of one or both heels. In my case, the pain was so severe I was mentally steeled to have surgery to repair it. I was that desperate for relief! To this day I don't know why my wife, who has known you for years, suggested that I go see you for this particular problem, but I did. It seemed weird to me because I thought all a chiropractor was good for was relieving back pain or neck pain. The pain in my entire foot had gotten so bad that I had to muster all my strength and pride to limp my way to your office. The rest is history! Dr. Beavers, can you explain in layman's terms what my problem was and how you fixed me?

Dr. Beavers: That's right. You were actually limping pretty badly when you came to my office that day. I distinctly remember that, and that you were in a great amount of pain. It didn't take me very long to figure out that the problem did not start in your foot, heel, or arch. It actually started way up high in your pelvis. Your pelvis was rotated, and your right hip was rotating as well, due to the muscles up in that hip flexor that had gotten too tight. And due to your hip rotation, your knee was also rotating, and [the issue] was working its way all the way down to your ankle and foot. So, not only did I have to change the alignment over time of how you were walking on that foot and ankle, which had shortened that plantar facia, which became inflamed on you, I had to correct the misalignment way up high in your pelvis. If I hadn't done that, whatever treatment I did wouldn't have lasted. Despite the work I did, your foot pain would have kept recurring due to the misalignment in your hip and pelvis.

LaRue: As Dr. Beavers said, the source of my problem was much higher up than my painful heel that I was sure needed surgery. Following my adjustment, I had significant relief in my heel. That's when, as I stood there in amazement, you sang that cute little song about how "chiropractic works!"

Dr. Beavers: It does [laughing], and I always tell my patients, "Guess what, where you're having pain is not where it starts most of the time. Where you're feeling the pain is the residual problem, which is starting from somewhere else." As chiropractors, we're trained to be detectives to figure out what's the source, what's the actual cause of the problem, because nine times out of ten it doesn't stem from where your pain is.

LaRue: Absolutely. And after you treated me, I decided to do some research because it was amazing to me that chiropractic really did work in my case, and I needed to better understand it. When it came to spinal adjustments, one of the things that helped me to understand chiropractic better was the analogy you gave me of an electrician, and how current has difficulty traveling through a crimped wire. Can you expound on that analogy?

Dr. Beavers: Yes, that's a great analogy I love to use. The spinal cord is a continuation of the brain stem and runs down through the spine. Branching off of that are the nerves at every single level of your spine. Those nerves send an electrical current to all the different systems of your body—whether it be your hearing, your sense of taste, your sense of smell, your heart, the function of your digestive system. All of that. I've had patients who have come in with ringing in their ears that wasn't the initial reason for the visit. But after I've treated them for their upper neck pain, they will say, "Oh, my gosh! I used to have this really bad ringing in my ears, and I don't have that anymore!"

Also, I have a longtime patient whom you know well because you've worked with her for years, who first came to me for chiropractic treatment. As it turns out, she was suffering from significant hearing loss—so much so that when she was in the office, she would shout at the top of her lungs because she couldn't hear herself. But now that she's been under a course of care with me for a couple of years, the improvement in her hearing is amazing! She doesn't shout anymore, and I no longer have to quiet her down so that other patients aren't disturbed. Although it's better when she can look right at you so that she can read your lips, she can carry on a conversation at a normal voice level now. I see her as my poster child for improvement with chiropractic care. I'd say her hearing improved at least 50 percent with chiropractic care, for sure!

LaRue: That's so amazing! I wrote about our dear Raina and her husband Alan in Chapter 6. That's such a good example to our readers of the benefits of chiropractic care, especially when it becomes a regular part of your health regimen. I'm a living testimony myself, coming from the unenlightened into the light! By the way, the plantar fasciitis you treated years ago is 100 percent healed—not even a hint of a problem—and I still spend lots of time on my feet during workouts and in the kitchen. Of course, I do make sure to get treatments at least twice a year to keep my body flexible and my organs working optimally. Which brings me to another point.

As a diabetes educator, I focus on diabetes self-management and care with any clients I have that live with diabetes. In my research, I've come across countless articles and studies that credit chiropractic care for helping to improve the processing of blood sugar through the pancreas. Because of that, I make sure that all my clients living with diabetes get a chiropractic adjustment at least twice a year.

DR. BEAVERS: Absolutely! That's a perfect example of how chiropractic care can benefit the various systems of the body. Your specialty in diabetes management highlights the fact that a middle-back adjustment can help our clients in significant ways, for sure.

LARUE: While doing research on this book, I came across some information that perhaps you don't know about. The Spanish flu epidemic of 1918 to 1920 infected over 500 million people—about a third of the world's population at the time. During the peak of the pandemic, thousands of infected people were simply left to die in various medical facilities, given no hope for survival by Western-medicine practitioners. It was then that chiropractors stepped up to treat thousands of those patients, most of whom survived because of their ongoing treatments.

DR. BEAVERS: Actually, I had heard of that. It's an amazing story and I'm so glad to learn that you shared it in your book.

LARUE: I have one final point I want to discuss with you. It's about something that many of us are left with in this post-pandemic era. Stress. For a number of reasons, stress is one of those things that we don't pay enough attention to, but it's a major factor in a number of health issues, especially for men. Mother Nature's cruel little trick played on men is that we tend to store the majority of our excess body fat in our belly, which is very unhealthy because that visceral fat compacts our internal organs and greatly increases our risk for a number of diseases, including obesity. When it comes to stress, you and I both know that unmanaged stress releases more cortisol, the fat-blocking hormone that prevents humans from releasing stored fat around their middle, no matter how much they exercise or diet. Can chiropractic care aid in relieving stress in the body?

DR. BEAVERS: If your sympathetic nervous system is always turned on, it's definitely going to release a lot of cortisol. And when you have all that excess cortisol in your body, things are going to happen as you described. Getting that nervous system to calm down [with a chiropractic adjustment] can definitely help. There are ways to stimulate the sympathetic nervous system with an adjustment, and there are ways to calm it down. You can do both things with an adjustment, depending on what the patient's needs are.

LARUE: This is definitely a man cave issue, because men like to suppress their feelings, hide their stress, and act like they've got everything under control, and that exacerbates the problem with stress. It's not being managed—it's simply being buried—and men don't let on that they are struggling because they don't want to let on that they need help, as though it's a sign of weakness. The irritability, anger, and moodiness sometimes spill over into toxic masculinity because men feel their masculinity being threatened. That's why I go to great lengths to encourage men to bring others into their man cave—for instance, a trusted friend, a relative, or even their health practitioner. A lot of deception and dishonesty takes place when men finally do go to see a doctor. That limits the opportunity to make progress towards healing.

DR. BEAVERS: I agree. A lot of patients after they get a chiropractic adjustment, when they come back for their next visit, they tell how much better they are sleeping, or how much calmer they feel since getting adjusted. And I'll be honest, hearing that is like icing on the cake for me—to know that what I've done for them makes such a big difference in their life. Especially when they didn't come in initially to address that problem, but it was a comment they made after having an adjustment.

LARUE: Health, nutrition, and wellness are hallmarks of both our professions, and helping our clients attain that takes a lot of detective work. Both of us have to do an initial health assessment when we see a patient, and I notice a particular trait we have that is identical. You are the consummate detective, always looking for clues, indications, or information that can help you in your treatment. And to a larger point, striving for wellness in all areas of the human body is an important part of the chiropractic world. Having the privilege of working in your clinic afforded me the opportunity to see how there was more concern for all aspects of health, nutrition, and wellness on behalf of your patients than one might see in a regular doctor's office.

DR. BEAVERS: For sure! And to help accomplish that goal I have the pleasure of having you as my health coach, where my patients get to take advantage of having that service available to them. Health and nutrition are key to supplementing the body's nervous system because you've got to eat well, you've got to exercise, and you've got to stretch. All those things feed and nourish the body, and also calm the body. It's all important.

LARUE: Dr. Beavers, we could certainly go on for quite a while talking about all things health related, but I believe we've hit a number of high points that my readers will be able to reflect on and take away from our discussion. And I'm sure that my readers will think a second time about assuming wrongly that a chiropractor is only good or necessary when you have some type of neck or back strain. I'm so glad I followed my wife's example and came to you when I did, or I would probably still be limping around like an old man on a bad wheel. Thank you for your time!

About the Author

LaRue Palmer is a career chef who decided to channel his spiritual gift for helping others into a career that is also a ministry. Leaving behind a successful career in Business Affairs in the Entertainment Industry, he returned to college and completed the degree he had started forty years prior. He earned his Bachelor of Science from Biola University, in Organizational Leadership, then embarked on a new career in culinary. He had a meteoric rise through the ranks, ranging from being a personal chef, to starting his own catering business, to working in the assisted-living industry as a food-service director. From there, he moved into fine dining at some of the top restaurants in Los Angeles, which landed him at SpaceX, where he helped open a state-of-the-art kitchen and corporate restaurant for Elon Musk.

His time at SpaceX afforded him the opportunity to attend the famous Integrative Institute of Nutrition, where he was certified, as well as getting certified as a Diabetes Education Specialist. He conceived the idea of launching a corporate health division at SpaceX, but decided instead to accept an offer to join Chiro-Integrative Health in Beverly Hills, where he could establish himself independently. The career change set him on a new course as a men's health advocate, which has become his sweet spot. LaRue has made numerous appearances on KTLA morning news and does frequent speaking engagements. He lives in Los Angeles, California, with his wife Ziva and daughter Arielle and their cats Zoey and Elliott.

Can You Help?

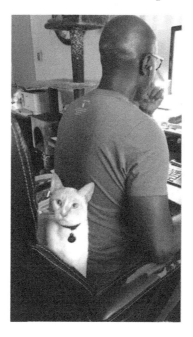

Thank You for Reading My Book!

I really appreciate all of your feedback, and I love hearing what you have to say.

I need your input to make the next version of this book and my future books better.

Please leave me an honest review on Amazon, letting me know what you thought of the book.

Thanks so much!

Endnotes

[1] "Provisional COVID-19 Deaths by Sex and Age," https://data.cdc.gov/NCHS/Provisional-COVID-19-Deaths-by-Sex-and-Age/9bhg-hcku/data.

[2] "Leading Causes of Death - Males - All races and origins - United States, 2016," https://www.cdc.gov/healthequity/lcod/men/2016/all-races-origins/index.htm.

[3] Philip Zimbardo, TED talks, Ted^xRawaRiverSalon, "Why Boys Are Failing?" https://www.youtube.com/watch?v=sgAu1i6aChs.

[4] Quote from neuroscientist Annaliese Beery, Smith College, Northampton, Maine, "who has been calling for researchers to address sex differences since 2009, and whose work was part of a larger movement that led to the NIH mandate," in Brooke Borel, "Of Mice and Men," https://www.spectrumnews.org/features/deep-dive/of-mice-and-women/.

[5] Kenia Pedrosa Nunes, Hicham Labazi, and R. Clinton Webb, "New Insights into Hypertension-associated Erectile Dysfunction," *Current Opinion in Nephrology and Hypertension* 2012: 21(2):163–170, doi: 10.1097/MNH.0b013e32835021bd.

[6] "Man Cave Health & Mount Sinai Health System," https://www.youtube.com/watch?v=9pKtKWmjiK8.

[7] National Center for Chronic Disease Prevention and Health Promotion (NCCDPHP), "Health and Economic Costs of Chronic Diseases, https://www.cdc.gov/chronicdisease/about/costs/index.htm.

[8] "Table 1. Deaths Involving Coronavirus Disease 2019 (COVID-19), Pneumonia, and Influenza Reported to NCHS by Time Period, Jurisdiction of Occurrence, Sex, and Age-group," https://www.cdc.gov/healthequity/lcod/men/2016/all-races-origins/index.htm.

[9] Ken Branson, *Rutgers Today*, March 23, 2016, "The Tougher Men Think They Are, the Less Likely They Are to Be Honest with Doctors," https://www.rutgers.edu/news/tougher-men-think-they-are-less-likely-they-are-be-honest-doctors. Original article (requires log-in): Mary S. Himmelstein and Diana T.

Sanchez, "Masculinity Impediments: Internalized Masculinity Contributes to Healthcare Avoidance in Men and Women," first published Oct. 7, 2014, *Journal of Health Psychology*, https://doi.org/10.1177/1359105314551623.

[10] The HUEman Races, "Popeye's Chicken Car Accident," https://www.youtube.com/watch?v=nkJKkltIo7A.

[11] WBAL-TV 11 Baltimore, "Man Fatally Stabbed at Popeye's after Cutting in Line," https://www.youtube.com/watch?v=W05V2PG1JJg; "Suspect Arrested in Deadly Stabbing of Customer Outside of Popeye's in Maryland," wusa9, https://www.wusa9.com/article/news/local/maryland/popeyes-stabbing-suspect-wanted/65-6b50765a-4ce7-44eb-9f9e-7cfaff49f550.

[12] Cleveland Clinic Mercy Hospital, "42 % of Americans Are Vitamin D Deficient. Are You Among Them?" https://www.cantonmercy.org/healthchat/42-percent-of-americans-are-vitamin-d-deficient/.

[13] Walter R. Rhodes, *The Official History of Chiropractic in Texas*, excerpts from Chapter 6 by Dan Murphy, as posted on "1918 Influenza Epidemic and Chiropractic Care," https://planetc1.com/1918-influenza-epidemic-and-chiropractic-care.

Made in the USA
Columbia, SC
20 December 2021

51961310R00098